Lectures on the

Methodology of
Clinical Research

Lectures on the

Methodology of Clinical Research

MAX HAMILTON

M.D., F.R.C.P., F.R.C.Psych., F.B.Ps.S.

Nuffield Professor of Psychiatry, University of Leeds

Hon. Consultant Psychiatrist, General Infirmary at Leeds; St. James's (University) Hospital, Leeds and Stanley Royd Hospital, Wakefield

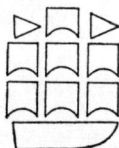

CHURCHILL LIVINGSTONE

EDINBURGH AND LONDON 1974

CHURCHILL LIVINGSTONE
Medical Division of Longman Group Limited

Represented in the United States of America by
Longman Inc., New York, and by associated
companies, branches and representatives throughout
the world.

First published 1961
Second edition 1974
ISBN 0 443 01080 3
Library of Congress Catalog Card No. 73-89665
Printed in Great Britain

PREFACE TO THE SECOND EDITION

Books, like human beings, grow larger as they grow older: this is unfortunate, but it cannot be helped. This second edition is bigger than the first but the growth is a compromise between the need to keep it as small as possible and the request of many readers to add more material on the practical aspects of research and on statistical calculations. I know that I have omitted many important themes, but decisions had to be made and I can only hope that they have been the right ones. Fortunately, it has been possible to introduce some modern notions in statistics without adding further to the size of this edition and I would like to think that the changes have increased the book's value to beginners in research without adding to their burdens.

I would like to thank Mrs. Betty Barnes for the typing of the manuscript and also Dr. Ken Warren and Mr. Colin Pritchard who acted as " guinea pigs " and made some useful comments on the clarity of the text and some suggestions for the glossary. Finally, I would like to acknowledge the help given to me by my Assistant, Mrs. Joy M. Brierly, in the preparation of the manuscript, for the proof-reading and indexing and also for help with the calculations.

MAX HAMILTON

LEEDS, 1974

PREFACE TO THE FIRST EDITION

Medical post-graduates can constitute the toughest audiences that a lecturer may meet. It is my experience that they are of high ability, have a good background of science, and because of their training in the art of interviewing patients, tend not to be over-awed by a lecturer. I am sure that this contributes to their sophisticated and even cynical attitude to lectures and lecturers. In direct contrast to this is their rather naïve attitude which tends to put at opposite poles the science of medicine, by which is implied laboratory work and diagnostic machinery, and the art of medicine, which is essentially regarded as clinical judgement, based on experience. If this remark seems exaggerated, it will be amply confirmed by a perusal of medical journals, wherein will be found articles and lectures in which the art of medicine is counterposed to the science. But there can be no doubt that clinical practice needs much more science than it has had heretofore. It is not sufficient for the clinician to rely on his empirical "experience" and ability to understand the patient as a human being, leaving the "science" to specialists and technicians. This can lead to one end only: the disappearance of the clinician (who sees the patient as a whole and treats him as a person), and his replacement by a group of specialists, who are interested primarily in their speciality.

It is on the basis of this opinion and with this particular audience in mind that I designed this set of lectures and gave them first in 1953. The lectures have been repeated annually, and among those who have attended regularly have been physicians, surgeons, obstetricians, anaesthetists, clinical pathologists and psychiatrists. That I have been able to retain their interest is sufficient proof that the lectures were useful. On a number of occasions I have been asked to publish these lectures, but have refrained from doing so on the grounds that there were many good books already available on the subject.

Recently I have been "going through the literature" and have been surprised how many books there were, and how very good they were. It is true that the number that deals directly with problems of clinical medicine is small, and it can be said of many of them that they are very much concerned with statistics as such

vii

and the details of computation. Books on the design of experiments also tend to be difficult. Perhaps there is room for a small book, one that is concerned primarily with clinical problems and concentrates on the logic and principles of the application of science to clinical research.

A word of explanation for the title: of course, these "lectures" are not transcriptions of the lectures as given. The conversational and colloquial style of speech appropriate to a small audience is quite unsuited for writing. So also are those pleasantries and asides which give an audience a moment's rest and renew its concentration. The questions and discussions which interrupt a lecture, and which are so important for making the hearers active participants in the process of learning instead of mere passive recipients of information, have perforce been omitted. Nevertheless, there are good reasons for retaining the form of " lectures ". The first is that it is made clear that this work is not intended to compete with the many excellent text-books. Lectures should never attempt to do what can be done by a text-book; their prime function is to give students help and guidance in the use of text-books. The second reason is that thereby I can retain the original " spiral structure " of the lectures: the return, again and again, to the same themes, but each time at a higher level. Such a structure is particularly suited to an elementary course of lectures, but is inappropriate in a book which will be used not only for instruction but for continued reference.

For any merits that this book possesses, I have to thank two persons in particular. First, Emeritus Professor Sir Cyril Burt, of the Department of Psychology, University College, London, for not only did he introduce me to scientific method, but he was the first of my teachers to demand high standards of me. Second, Dr. Ardie Lubin, of the Walter Reed Army Institute of Research, Washington, D.C., whose eminent use of the Socratic method has forced me to try to think clearly. There are passages in this book which remind me of particular sessions with him, stimulating, exciting, but very strenuous. I would also like to thank Miss M. Knott for her care in the preparation of the script and help with the index, and Miss E. Read, B.A., Librarian of the Leeds Medical School, for help in finding some of the references.

MAX HAMILTON

WAKEFIELD, 1961

Contents

ix

Introduction: Structure of a Research Project

These lectures are entitled ' Lectures on the Methodology of Clinical Research '. Let me explain this. In the course of these lectures I am going to give an account of the underlying principles and methods of thinking involved in doing clinical research. I shall try to explain how one formulates a clear question and then designs an investigation to obtain an answer. This means, in practice, designing a procedure for yielding appropriate data and drawing inferences from them. This, because of the variability of biological material, requires a statistical analysis. I shall try to show that the techniques of statistical analysis are merely a particular way of drawing inferences from data. To the beginner, this appears to be a formidable task but I hope to demonstrate that the essence of the designing of clinical investigations and the analysis of the resulting data is a comprehensible logical process.

It is an interesting experience to examine a very old copy of a medical journal: the general appearance is quaint and even amusing. For example, that very respected British medical journal, *The Lancet*, first came out in pocket magazine size—diminutive medical journals are not at all a new idea—and its contents, to the modern reader, are astonishing, to say the least. They consist very much of medical news and accounts and reports of lectures, the latter containing a surprising amount of personal anecdotes. There is sometimes a vague air of the newspaper advertisement about these lectures ' I did the following and the patient was cured '.

The contents of a recent number of a general medical journal are very different indeed. Most of the material in the journal is a description of original research work, a good deal of which consists of biochemical, physical and chemical investigations, with a sprinkle of clinical ones. Of the last group, the great majority consist of ' clinical trials '. These consist of carefully planned investigations to evaluate a treatment and the result is usually expressed in statistical terms. Many others are concerned with prognosis and the determination of prognostic criteria. Others are concerned with refinements of diagnostic techniques. All of these papers use statistics to describe their results, even if these are at the lowest level of mere proportions or percentages. The emphasis is on the use of scientific methods for the increase of knowledge, and the change in these medical journals reflects an important change in medicine.

In the past century, the art of medicine has changed largely from a traditional craft to an applied science. All of us who are engaged in the practice of medicine have a duty to our patients, to do the best we can for them, and this requires not only that we should understand the new developments but also to some extent that we should contribute to them. For the best way of understanding what is new in medicine is to take part in it. It is for this reason that so many young doctors are now enthusiastically interested in or trying to do research. The same can be said for associated professions, e.g. social workers and nurses.

Motives for Research

It is easy to be very cynical about this and to believe that the only reason why doctors, particularly young ones, are engaged in research or express an interest or an enthusiasm for it, is that they do so in order to advance themselves in their professions. The interest is not in research but merely in ' getting on '. This sort of opinion, it seems to me, is not so much cynical as silly. All young doctors have to make their way, and they do so by securing the approval of the older and more senior members of their profession. They do this by conforming to what is regarded as the right and proper way of doing things. When the proper way is the practice of medicine that is what they do; and when it is research, they do that. In America, if one wishes to become a Professor of Psychiatry, almost invariably it is necessary to undergo psycho-analysis; so young psychiatrists get themselves psycho-analysed. In other countries this is a very undesirable thing to do, so they don't. In the 17th century, the aspiring English physician paid a visit to Italy, in the 19th he went to Germany and nowadays he goes to the United States.

The motives for research are a personal matter and of little concern to others. What matters is the result, the research itself. There are only two kinds of research, not those with good or bad motives, but just those that are good or bad. It is true that many doctors express a desire to do research only because they think that if they publish enough papers they will get better jobs. It seems to me that this could be as good a reason for doing research as any, but the man who boasts of a long list of second rate papers concerned with trivial matters, condemns himself in the eyes of his peers. If he wants to make a name for himself he can best do so by trying to do good research.

There is also another good reason for trying to do good research. There is no point in doing research unless it is published. The number of papers offered to journals is steadily increasing. It is increasing, believe it or not, even faster than the number of journals and this means that the pressure on editors is rising. The selection of papers for publication therefore becomes steadily more intense. If you want your paper to be published, it had better be a good one. I won't discuss other motives, such as the satisfaction obtained from doing good work and from playing one's part in the advancement of medicine. Surely these go without saying.

Even if we are not likely to be involved in research, we still have to understand what it is all about. We are all ' consumers ' of research, even if we are not producers. At the best, we want to keep up-to-date with judgment and discrimination. At the worst, we shall quickly find that the investigations and treatments we order for our patients cease to be available.

Research and Clinical Practice

It is often said that good clinical practice is incompatible with research, or at least that the attitude of the clinician prevents him from taking part in clinical research. I disagree with this completely. No clinician can rest satisfied with present-day therapies. Every one concerned with sick people is delighted when a patient recovers and even more so when he has good reason to believe that it is his intervention which has produced the recovery; but that is not enough, he should also worry about the failures of treatment and these should be his constant preoccupation. The aim of medicine is, ideally, to prevent disease and when this fails, to cure it; but from where does the knowledge for this come? Everyone will agree that for proper diagnosis and treatment, a good clinical history is fundamental. Surely this provides the data for hypotheses concerning the causation of the patient's illness? The clinician cannot shut his eyes to this. Even at this most basic level, good clinical practice provides the data for research.

A doctor should give his patient the best treatment that he can. But what is the best? Presumably it means the treatment which will give the best result for the particular patient. How can this be known without careful study of the factors in the patients' condition and in their history and background which are related to the outcome of a particular treatment. Here again is the basic material for clinical research.

It is a tradition of medicine that doctors should try to use a new treatment if there is evidence which suggests that it is better than the old. But what is evidence? Traditionally, it is the say-so of ' authorities ', but we know only too well from the history of medicine that this is just as likely to lead to the introduction of useless and even harmful remedies as lead to good ones. When the physician tries a new remedy, surely it is worth his while to try to collect the evidence that will demonstrate its superiority to the old treament. The cautious physician sticks to the old and may thereby find himself depriving his patients of the benefits of the new. The enthusiast swings over to the new and may find himself exposing his patients to dangers. Neither of them can contribute to new knowledge and therefore to improve our methods of treatment. It is the intermediate approach which does so. A gradual change over from the old treatment to the new means that some patients are receiving the old treatment and some the new and this is clearly the basis of the modern clinical experiment with its control series. Such a cautious approach can be carried out even when a physician is trying a new treatment for the first time. Obviously he will try it on those patients who have failed to respond to traditional treatment. In doing so, he does not deprive them of the full benefits of what is already known and yet gives them a second chance to benefit. Once the physician has gained experience with this treatment and finds that it is not unsatisfactory he can then extend its use by giving it to those patients whom he would expect to be failures of treatment. The third stage is obvious, when he starts to give it to the general run of patients but always remembering to compare the new with the old in proper fashion.

The Structure of a Research Project

A good way to begin is to consider the structure of a published paper describing a piece of research. If you understand this clearly it will also help you when you come to write up your own reports.

It is often complained of such papers that they do not really give an account of how the work was carried out. There is no description of the struggle to define the questions, to develop a satisfactory method of investigation and to overcome the practical difficulties that were met. There is nothing about the false starts and the trails that led nowhere. There is a good reason for this: such matters are largely of personal interest. Perhaps the biographer of the researcher, or the historian, might be interested in them. The purpose of a scientific report is to give the reader information of two kinds. The first is concerned with the actual findings and the second with the background which enables the reader to evaluate them.

A research paper can be divided into six sections. They are:

1. Review of the Literature.
2. Statement of the problem.
3. The method of investigation.
4. The results and the conclusions.
5. Discussion of the results.
6. Summary.

REVIEW OF THE LITERATURE

When you start to read a paper, having first read the title, you will at least have some notion of what it is going to be about. The purpose of the review of the literature is to give detailed information about the subject. It will tell you what has been done in that field of study and also, ideally, it will tell you what has *not* been done. It will give an account of the background of the subject and will do all this in a critical fashion. In other words, the author will explain the value of the work that has been done, describing those researches which have achieved something and those which are inadequate in the way they have been carried out, and giving the evidence to demonstrate this. Above all, the review of the literature should explain to you why the subject *matters*. Ideally, when you have finished reading the review of the literature you will not only have a fair notion of what the problem is all about but what will be the nature of the investigation to be described in the paper and why it should have been undertaken.

I am always very suspicious of the review of the literature which is uninformative and which gives a large number of references. ' The factors affecting the concentration of this constituent of the blood have been investigated on a number of occasions (1), (3), (5),

(7), (9), (11). Some of these findings have been accepted (4), (6), (8), and others have not been confirmed, (10), (12), (13), (14).' When I read this sort of drivel I have a strong belief that the writer has not actually read the works to which he refers, but has merely copied out the names from some other paper, and I will need a good deal of evidence to convince me that this is not so. Sometimes, such lists of papers are amplified by brief statements about their contents, but bitter experience has taught me that such descriptions can be misleading. Careful examination of the papers referred to has sometimes shown me that the writer referring to them has read only the summary, because the summary differs from the content of the paper. I remember one paper in particular that was referred to repeatedly for many years and was stated to have proved that the response of some patients to psychotropic drugs depended upon their environmental circumstances. Careful reading of the paper itself demonstrated only too clearly that the authors had considered that this might be a possibility but one which did not even arise from the data in the paper. The function of the review of the literature is to inform the reader rather than to advertise the writer.

At this point I would like to mention that the structure of a paper published in a journal is exactly the same as the structure of a thesis for a higher degree. The essential difference is simply the amount of space available. The investigator who writes a paper for publication in a journal will generally cut it down to an irreducible minimum; if he doesn't the Editor will. When an investigator writes a thesis he does not have to worry about considerations of space. He can afford to spread himself and to discuss matters in detail. This applies particularly to the review of the literature. So, for those of you who are contemplating doing a piece of research for a thesis, I would like to give you some advice concerning the writing-up.

When you write the review of the literature, you should give plenty of quotations and when you give an opinion or an evaluation of a particular piece of work, you should always back it with the evidence required. You should give your reader all the information necessary for him to accept your conclusions about the content and the value of the paper. You should not hesitate to compliment or to criticize adversely any particular investigation. Fortunately, since most theses are not published, they can be considered as semi-private documents and you do not therefore need to worry about being tactful about bad work or a fear of the possibility of a libel action. Ideally, your reader should be given all the information required about the paper you are discussing. The only reason why he should need to go and look at the original paper itself is to check whether in fact you are telling the truth; certainly not because he cannot understand what you have written.

STATEMENT OF THE PROBLEM

If the review of the literature is adequate, then by the time the reader comes to the end he should know exactly what the problem is and have a shrewd idea of how it should be investigated. The simple statement of the problem makes this perfectly clear. There are two ways of describing the problem: either as a direct statement, e.g. ' This investigation is concerned with whether . . .', or in the form of a question. The purists prefer the latter form and with good reason. If you are going to put yourself to a good deal of trouble to collect data to answer a question, you might as well ask the question clearly at the beginning. Speaking personally, either way is equally good. All that matters is that the reader should be perfectly clear about the nature of the problem. There is one method of stating the problem which should *never* be used and that goes—' The following investigation was designed to disprove the null hypothesis that . . .' There was a fashion for this in psychological journals at one time and I could never understand how the Editors could pass this silliness. Incidentally, the statement of the problem should be accompanied by such definitions of terms that will clarify ambiguities and explain unfamiliar terms. I remember reading a paper on ' unstable angina ' which never condescended to explain what the term meant. In a journal of cardiology this would be acceptable, but this paper was in a general medical journal.

METHOD OF INVESTIGATION

The next part of the paper describes the method of investigation. Strictly speaking, this section of the paper should describe the whole procedure in complete detail. In practice, this is not possible and very often not really desirable. If standard tests, biochemical, physiological or psychological, are used, then there should be no need to describe these in detail. The readers can reasonably be expected to know what they are. At the most, a reference to the original descriptions should be sufficient. If non-standard or new tests are used these should be described in sufficient detail. If full details have already been given in a previous publication, these can be referred to but a good paper will, even in these circumstances, give some account of these new and relatively unknown tests. This is the sort of thing that the reader wants to know and the way in which it is done shows the judgment of the writer.

Then follows the design of the experiment and a description of the 'material' on which it was carried out. If it is a biochemical investigation carried out on bits of tissue, then the method of preparing them will be described. If it is an experiment on animals, then the type of animal will be defined. If the investigation is carried out on patients suffering from a given disorder, then the diagnosis will be given in sufficient detail to make clear to the reader what sort of illness it was. Furthermore, the type of patient should be described properly. What this means depends very much on circumstances but the essence of this description is that the group of patients on whom the investigation was carried out should be described in such a way that they are identifiable. The report of an investigation is, in a sense, an historical document. It describes what was done by the investigator and that is something that happened in the past. It is of interest to the reader chiefly because it serves as a guide to action in the future. If the paper describes the result of treatment, you will want to know whether this treatment is worth using and therefore you will want to know to what sort of patient it should be applied. If this is not given clearly in the paper then obviously the rest of the information in the paper is useless.

RESULTS

By the time you reach this point you may have come to the conclusion that the investigation was carried out so badly or so pointlessly that you are not interested at all in whatever results were obtained. In that case, you will pass on. If, however, you are still interested, you will now expect to read a description of what was found. The findings are generally expressed in statistical terms and these are of two kinds—descriptive statistics and evaluative statistics. The latter are the tests of significance and I shall describe them in detail later.

DISCUSSION AND SUMMARY

In the discussion, the author takes his results and puts them against the background which he has described in the first part of the paper. He considers in what way his findings are in agreement with those of others and in what way they differ and he goes on to consider what these resemblances and differences signify. If his findings have any relevance to theoretical problems, he will then go into this.

If the Editor of the journal has given the author sufficient space, he will then go on to consider the merits and demerits of his work. This has two aspects; the first is concerned with what has or has not been achieved, by his investigation; the second is concerned with the success or failure, in the sense of limitations, of the investigation. Finally, the author will then suggest in what way further work can develop from what he has done.

The summary is the first thing that the experienced reader will turn to when he has read the title of the paper, and for this reason it has become customary in recent years for the summary to be placed above the main body of the paper, with special emphasis on the results and some brief statement about the method. Although the summary should be brief, it should also be informative. There are few things I find more exasperating than the sort of summary which states ' an investigation into certain problems has been described and the results listed '. This is about as useful as a sick headache. The summary should be accurate and I regret to say that this is not always so. I never know whether to be amused or annoyed by this, but it is well you should remember it when you have need to look up references.

Summary

In this lecture I have given an account of the structure of a research report published in a medical journal. This structure is important not only because that is the way one should write a paper, but also because it reflects the structure and procedures of the research itself. It therefore gives, in outline, an introduction to the various stages of a research project.

The Stages of Experimentation: I

I shall start this lecture by considering the nature of experimentation. The experimental method essentially contains four stages. They are are as follows: Observation, Hypothesis, Experimentation and Induction. What I shall do is to go over these briefly and then, in subsequent lectures, I shall deal with each stage in detail and explain what I mean.

Observation

As you know teaching in medicine is traditionally very didactic. This is not entirely the fault of the teachers. The medical student is so acutely aware of the vast amount of factual material which he has to assimilate, that he is apt to become impatient and restless when his teachers take time off from pumping facts into him, to go into other matters. This is most unfortunate, because at the core of the scientific attitude is the constant awareness of the immensity of our ignorance. Science is a tremendous adventure of exploration, making the unknown known, bringing light into darkness and order into chaos. In medicine in particular, as in biology in general, we are always on the edge of the unknown. We can ask questions about any problem, no matter how simple or trivial it may seem, to which nobody knows the answers. Questions are everywhere and that is what research is for, to find answers to them. The research worker does not go around vaguely wondering and hoping that he will find something. We find answers only from our experience but this experience must be based on deliberate and careful observation of the world around us. This is the foundation of all research.

How does one set about it? This can be only partially systematized, for there is little one can say about it in the way of formulating any specific rules. In the first place one's ability to see what is going on and to understand it depends on a profound knowledge of the material one is observing, for it is not sufficient merely to see, one has to understand the meaning and significance of what is observed. For example, it is very important to recognize what is common and what is uncommon. In the world of medicine we had a great example of this remarkable ability in the person of Dr Parkes-Weber, the ' specialist in rare diseases '. This ability to recognize in the course of work that an unusual phenomenon is occurring and to see its significance, is dependent upon experience. I would like to emphasize this point: that only those who are dealing with the material in the course of clinical work, who are primarily clinicians, can recognize these qualities when they see them, and realize their significance. Clinical observation is the essence of this stage. The history of science is full of this.

I would like to spend many interesting hours giving you examples, but I shall have to content myself with only a few. Take the classic example in physiology of the attendant in Minkowski's laboratory who noticed that there were a lot of flies hanging around the urine of dogs who had been operated on. The story goes that he tasted the urine and found it to be sweet. He mentioned this to Minkowski who knew that they had had their pancreases removed. Now this was very acute observation, and it enabled Minkowski to demonstrate that removal of the pancreas produced the condition of diabetes mellitus. This was one of the first clues to the nature of diabetes and on the metabolism of sugar*. Another example of acute observation is that of Pasteur who, when working with crystals of tartaric acid, noticed that these were of two kinds which were mirror images of each other. I won't give you full details, but it was this discovery that laid the foundation for a completely new science—the science of stereochemistry. The point being that he looked at them, he noticed them and he used his brains also to consider what the observation meant. Let me give a third example. In the late nineteenth century Lord Rayleigh, the chemist, was doing an experiment, a very simple routine experiment. He was determining the atomic weight of nitrogen; simple enough, but a finicky job that required great accuracy. He noticed that when his nitrogen was obtained from the air its atomic weight was slightly greater than that derived from ammonium nitrite. This difference was in the third decimal place, in the fifth significant figure, but he knew that he had done these experiments very, very carefully indeed and they should not have differed by three or four points in the third decimal place. So he proceeded to investigate this discrepancy

---

* I have not been able to trace the origin of the story of Minkowski's discovery of the effect of pancreatectomy, but the version of the story given comes from Sir Charles Lovatt Evans, who had it from Starling.

and as a result he discovered (with Ramsay) argon, neon, krypton, xenon and helium, all the noble gases.

I do not have to tell you the story of Fleming and the penicillium, but we can be quite sure that this sort of accident has occurred many times in the history of bacteriology. The point of the story being not so much that Fleming had the accidental experience, his bacterial culture being contaminated by penicillium, but that he realized the significance of it. One has not only to notice what is going on and recognize the unusual but think about it as well. There are no rules for this and no simple way of doing it.

Again and again one sees this in the history of medicine, particularly related to the side actions of drugs. A classic example which is now, in a sense, commonplace, but when it came out was a brilliant example of this work, is the story of the discovery of the use of mandelic acid as a treatment for infections of the urinary tract. The story begins with the ancient belief that epilepsy was improved by fasting. This was investigated by Geyelin, who reported favourable results from this method of treatment. This led Wilder to consider whether the effect of fasting on epilepsy might be due to the ketonaemia which results from such fasts. He decided to produce a ketonaemia by giving his patients a ketogenic diet, and found that this treatment did in fact give good results. The next step was made by Helmholz, and I quote his words: 'A chance observation of a specimen of urine from a patient on the ketogenic diet for the treatment of epilepsy showed it to be clear and apparently unspoiled after standing in a warm room for about a week. It seemed possible that patients in ketosis excreted a bactericidal urine'. Helmholz demonstrated that the bactericidal action of the urine was not due to its acidity but it was not until over a decade later that it was shown by Fuller that the bactericidal power lay in the ketones in the urine, and especially p-hydroxybutyric acid. Unfortunately, the diet is unpleasant and difficult to maintain and, of course, the acids of ketosis could not be administered because they are metabolized too quickly. It was argued by Rosenheim that modifications of the molecule of the ketotic acids would slow down their metabolism, and that is how he introduced the mandelic acid treatment. I do not have to tell an audience which includes psychiatrists, the story of Chlorpromazine, which was originally used by anaesthetists to potentiate barbiturates. The anaesthetist noticed the strange effect it had on patients who seemed to develop, after they had received the Chlorpromazine, an attitude of indiffer-

ence to the operation which they were about to have, and even afterwards seemed to take the whole business rather casually. When the
French psychiatrists heard about this they seized on this point
immediately and now we have more phenothiazines than we can
cope with.

My last example of acute observation is the story of the mercurial diuretics. The diuretic effects of compounds of mercury was
observed by Alfred Vogl in Vienna in October 1919 when he was
using such a compound in the treatment of a non-oedematous girl
with congenital neurosyphilis. For a whole day after such injections the urinary output was more than trebled. Vogl followed this
up and showed that this was not an effect of the drug on a syphilitic
organ but was a general diuretic effect previously unrecognized.

I will conclude this section by summarizing my main points.
There are no set rules for human ingenuity and constructive thinking, but they must be firmly based on an intensive knowledge of the
background of ones' subject and an understanding of what one is
doing. You must look at your material, you cannot do research
second-hand by ordering others to do this, that or the other; you
must do it yourself. You must look at the material yourself and
look at it hard; examine it again and again and think about it; and
this needs time. You cannot plan these things and rush them
through. You must have time to look at your data, to consider
them and speculate about them. Speculation is one of the most
important things in research but there is no way of formalizing it.
If you are hoping to learn something about research, I can tell you
about techniques, the way to tackle problems etc., but I cannot tell
you how to think. That you must do yourselves.

Hypothesis

Observation has suggested an idea, or in popular speech, a
' hunch '. To convert the idea into a hypothesis which can be tested
by an experiment it is necessary to make it clear and specific. Whatever it may be, a new method of treatment or a new method of
investigation, or even a new theoretical concept, it will have to be
tried out. This means that one will have to devise some method of
making appropriate observation and then coming to conclusions on
the basis of the results.

Unfortunatey, too many people stop at this last stage. They write
it up and send it to the journals and then the real trouble starts,

because we poor souls have to read it and wonder whether it is worth the effort.

The formulation of hypotheses is a stage of research not nearly as difficult as the first one with which I have already dealt, since we have some rules of procedure. The first thing to remember about a hypothesis which is going to be tested by an experiment, is that it must not be a general statement: it has to be one which is specific in every one of its parts. For example, one may have some vague idea that clinical factors or diet may affect the secretion of the thyroid gland. I once toyed with the idea of investigating environmental factors which may influence recovery from depressive illness. Obviously, such ideas are far too vague to form the basis of an investigation; they have to be refined or narrowed down and this process forms the basis of the planning of the experiment. Of course, in medicine, we make good use of those 'experiments' which Nature provides for us. When a patient falls ill with pneumonia then, as physicians, we must do our best to try to help him recover. As scientists, we are interested in the nature of the processes which make him ill. For example, what is the nature of the changes in the body produced by the pneumococci in the lungs and how are they effected? But, when we have made observations in these experiments, 'natural' or designed, we then have to make inferences from them, and this can be very difficult and full of pitfalls.

Drawing Inferences from Data

I shall give three simple examples to illustrate these difficulties.

Example (*A*). Before the Second World War, pregnant women were given iron in ante-natal clinics and, as a result, the concentration of haemoglobin in their blood increased. It was concluded, therefore, that they were suffering from anaemia. Is this true? No, not necessarily. It may well be that giving iron to pregnant women will always increase the amount of haemoglobin in their blood, whether they are anaemic or not.

Example (*B*). A surgeon reports an 80 per cent five-year survival rate, using his operation for carcinoma of the cervix at stage 1. This is much better than the usual figures. He concludes that his operation is a great improvement on other methods and advocates its use, Is he right? The conclusion does not necessarily follow from the data. It may well be that the patients come to him at a much earlier stage of their disease than at other surgical centres.

These two examples that I have given illustrate something important. Strictly speaking, from a logical point of view, the results of an experiment give information about that experiment, and about that experiment only. But these result are used to make general inferences, and it is this that is the essential problem. Now let us have a look at these two examples that I gave. Consider example A. The inference from this example is about the nature of disease processes. Because the blood haemoglobin increased, it was assumed that the patient was suffering from anaemia. In example B, the information is used to make the following inference about other patients; if this treatment be used on other patients, then better results will be achieved than by using the other methods. It is the type and nature of such inferences from experiments which concern us here.

LOGIC

Let us consider techniques for drawing inferences. There are certain rules for this and these rules are the subject-matter of logic. Logic is generally described as falling into two kinds: (a) deductive and (b) inductive. The former is the first type of logic to have been developed systematically, and dates from the days of Ancient Greece. Everybody knows something about the elements, they have all heard about the syllogism and the methods of deducing conclusions from simple statements. Let us take the classical syllogism: All men are mortal; Socrates is a man, therefore Socrates is mortal. Again: All swans are birds: this is a swan, therefore it is a bird.

Let us consider an example that is a little nearer home. Consider the situation where a treatment has been devised for an ' invariably fatal disease '. Until the present we could always say: This disease is invariably fatal; this patient suffers from it, therefore he will die of it. A patient is now given the treatment and does not die. It is clear that this patient does not constitute an example of the general rule, or the general rule is inapplicable to the example. We can deal with this situation by dividing the general rule into two categories: treated and untreated cases. The general statement now becomes: this disease, in the absence of treatment, is invariably fatal. Since the patient we are concerned with, does not fall into this group, we cannot deduce that he is one of those who will die, or alternatively, we can decide that he is not one of those who will necessarily die of the disease. So far, this is a matter of simple logic.

The next step is not so simple. Since untreated patients die, and this patient received treatment, it is easy to say that the patients did not die *because* of the treatment. In the way I have put it, it is clear that the conclusion does not follow from the premises, something extra has been introduced; but there is another difficulty. The statement that the disease in invariably fatal is not a definition, it is an *induction* derived from observation of the patients who have suffered from the disease, or, as the logician would put it, by observation of the members of the class. Such an induction can be made with certainty only after observation of all members of the class, and we have not observed all the patients who will suffer from the disease in the future. Unfortunately, past experience is no guarantee of the future. Although the disease has been invariably fatal in the past we have no proof that it will be so in the future. This is true of all our experience: the future is always, to some extent, uncertain.

From what I have just said, the distinction between deduction and induction is not always clear, although it is generally useful to think of deduction as the method of applying a general rule to a particular instance, and induction as the drawing of general conclusions from particular examples. In logical terms, we consider members of a class and make inferences about the class. Such inferences are always uncertain unless we can observe all the members of that class. From our point of view, one of the most important kinds of induction is the statistical kind, whereby we draw conclusions about a ' population ' from the ' sample ' that we have before us. I may add here that although our inferences may be uncertain, this uncertainty can be given a completely rigorous expression.

Deduction and Induction

Consider now example C and the conclusions we can draw by deductive and inductive logic. A sack contains 100 potatoes. We draw 20 of them at random and we observe they are of different sizes; we weigh them all together and find they come to 10 pounds. What can we infer from this simple observation? Deductively we can infer the following: As 20 of the potatoes weigh 10 pounds we can be sure that the total weight of the potatoes is more than ten pounds, since the other potatoes, being material objects, must have some weight. Furthermore, since the 20 potatoes that we have weigh ten pounds and the total number is 100 we know that the average weight of the potatoes must be greater than one-tenth of a pound, 10 pounds divided by 100. Consider the three statements. There are 100 potatoes, some of them weigh ten pounds, the average weight must be over one-tenth of a pound. Although there are three statements here, there are only two completely independent items of information. Given any two of the statements you can always extract information about the third without difficulty, and you will agree that the information is not very helpful.

What can be inferred by the second method, of induction? We have drawn 20 potatoes at random. They are of different sizes and they weigh ten pounds; their average weight is therefore half a pound. Inductively we can state that the average weight of all the potatoes is about half a pound and therefore very probably the sack weighs about fifty pounds, but we can't be certain. It's a good guess, if you like. This is the difference between deductive and inductive logic or thinking. At this point I must quote R. A. Fisher: ' New knowledge comes from experience by inductive inference and is the only way from which it can come '. Discussions on logic and the problems of drawing inferences from data are not mere intellectual amusements.

I am now going to put a question to you and I would like you to think carefully about the answer before you go on. I would suggest that you might even write down the answer or answers and compare them with what I say afterwards. If I give a patient a treatment and he recovers, what conclusions can I draw from the result of the ' experiment '? None, really, but if you insist on some sort of inference, then I can say that the patients do not invariably die from this disorder. If you prefer to think in terms of treatment, then I can say that I can conclude from this result that the treatment does not invariably kill the patients! Either way, the inference is so trivial that you can understand why I say that, for practical purposes, no conclusion can be drawn from a single case.

Let us go one step further and say that I do the experiment on a group of patients; now I find that 70 per cent have recovered. Can I draw any inferences from this? If you think about it carefully, you will see that even here it is not possible to draw any conclusions that are of any practical value. If, for example, the recovery rate for this disorder was 70 per cent even when untreated, then clearly my results show that the treatment is of no effect. If the recovery rate was considerably less than 70 per cent, then obviously it would be legitimate to consider that the treatment had improved the recovery rate; but if the recovery rate were normally much higher than 70 per cent, then one might infer that the treatment was, in fact, harming the patients and increasing the mortality. Unless I have some background information with which I can compare my present results, then I can draw no useful conclusions. The need for such background data with which one makes comparisons is just as important even in circumstances where they are not so obvious. Consider the physiologist who stimulates some part of the brain of an animal and shows that in consequence there is a rise in blood pressure. To make quite certain, he repeats the stimulation, and each time he produces an increase in blood pressure. He therefore concludes that it is the stimulation of this particular area of the brain which gives rise to an increase in the blood pressure. This pre-supposes that the rise of blood pressure disappeared and the blood pressure returned to normal after an interval and before the next stimulation. If this did not happen, then repeated stimulation would not produce the same effect as a single one. Either the effect of each successive stimulation would diminish until finally there was no effect, or else the animal would be killed. Either way, the effect of repeated stimulation would not be the same as that of a single stimulation and one would have to be very careful about drawing inferences from the results of this experiment. The assumption that the animal returns to its normal state after each stimulation is equivalent to having knowledge of the background state to which I have already referred. If we give a ' treatment ' and make observations before, during and after, then valid conclusions about the effects of the treatment can be made only if it can be demonstrated that the state ' after ' is the same as the state ' before '. If this is not so, then we must devise other methods for determining the ' background '.

Suppose an experimental cardiologist wishes to evaluate a new design for an artificial valve. Presumably, he will start by inserting it into the heart of an animal and then measuring how much the circulation is impaired thereby. In the present state of the art, no artificial valve can be expected to function as well as a natural one. Having made the measurements, is he now in a position to say what accounted for the deterioration in the circulation? Of course not, since it is obvious that such deterioration could be attributed to the effects of the anaesthetic or to the surgical interference with the heart. It is not unreasonable to assume that if the investigator waits long enough then the effects of the anaesthetic will wear off, but he still cannot differentiate between the effects of surgical operation on the heart and the effects of the substitution of the valve. Clearly he will have to do something special in order to determine this and this something special is an experiment.

Experimentation

The purpose of an experiment is to produce data from which it is possible to draw appropriate conclusions. The experiment must therefore be so designed that it is possible to draw valid conclusions. As R. A. Fisher said ' experimental observations are only experience carefully planned in advance and designed to form a secure basis of knowledge '. The great experimental physiologist Claude Bernard also emphasized the importance of experience in the form of planned experimentation. Knowledge, he declared, ' is always gained by virtue of precise reasoning based on an idea born of observation and controlled by experiment '. (You will notice how similar are the quotations from the two scientists, in themselves so unlike.)

How do you set about designing an experiment? First of all, you have to remember that the criteria of good experiments vary in time and place. An experiment arises from the existing body of knowledge to test hypotheses and theories arising from that knowledge, and on the basis of the experiments, these theories are appropriately modified and reformulated. Every experiment arises from the existing body of knowledge and those that are done now differ from those that were done in the past and will differ from those that will be done in the future.

Designing an experiment in order to draw valid conclusions implies that these conclusions will be based on the evidence of the experiment. This is absolutely fundamental in our notions of the nature of experiments; they must provide the evidence for their interpretation and this interpretation must depend solely on the data provided by them; in other words, the experiments must be self-contained. It is this which determines the difference between mere statistical observations and those which are collected in accordance with a clearly conceived plan.

Summary

The process of clinical investigation goes through a number of stages, of which the first is in many ways the most important. This is the stage of observing and recognizing that there is a phenomenon which needs investigation. The next stage is that of formulating a specific hypothesis which is suitable for testing by means of an experiment. The experiment must be designed in such a way that valid conclusions can be drawn from it. The validity depends not only on the design of the experiment but also on the proper use of logical induction.

REFERENCES

BERNARD, Claude (1865). *An Introduction to the Study of Experimental Medicine*, p. 12. New York: Dover Publications (1957).

DELAY, J. & DENIKER, P. (1952). 38 cas de psychoses traitees par la cure prolongee et continue de 4560 R.P. *Congrès Psychiatria neurologia*, pp. 503-513. Luxembourg: Longue Francais.

FLEMING, A. (1929). On antibacterial action of cultures of penicillium with special reference to their use in isolation of B. influenzae. *British Journal of Experimental Pathology*, **10**, 226-236.

FISHER, Sir Ronald A. (1935). *The Design of Experiments*, 6th edn, pp. 7, 18. Edinburgh: Oliver & Boyd.

FULLER, A. T. (1933). Ketogenic diet nature of bactericidal agent *Lancet*, **i**, 855-856.

GEYELIN, H. R. (1921). Fasting as a method for treating epilepsy. *Medical Record (New York)*, **99**, 1037-1039.

HELMHOLZ, H. F. (1931). The ketogenic diet in the treatment of pyuria of children with anomalies of the urinary tract. *Proceedings of the Mayo Clinic*, **6**, 609-613.

LABORIT, H., HUGUENARD, P. & ALLUAUME, R. (1952). Un nouveau stabilisateur vegetatif (le 4560 PR). *Presse médicale*, **60**, 206-208.

MINKOWSKI, O. & VON MEHRING, J. (1889). De l'extirpation du pancreas chez les animaux et du diabete experimental. *Semaine médicale*, **9**, 175-176.

MINKOWSKI, O. (1893). Untersuchung uber den Diabetesmellitus nach Extirpation des Pankreas. *Archiv für experimentelle Pathologie und Pharmakologie*, **31**, 85-189.

RAYLEIGH, Lord (1893). On the densities of the principal gases. *Proceedings of the Royal Society*, **53**, 146.

RAYLEIGH, Lord (1894). On an anomaly encountered in determinations of the density of nitrogen gas. *Proceedings of the Royal Society*, **55**, 340-344.

RAYLEIGH, Lord & RAMSAY, W. (1895). Argon, a new constituent of the atmosphere. *Philosophical Transactions (A)*, **186**, 187-241.

ROSENHEIM, M. L. (1935). Mandelic acid in the treatment of urinary infections. *Lancet*, **i**, 1032-1037.

VALLERY-RADOT, Rene (1911). *The Life of Pasteur*. English Trans. London, p. 38. (Original Paris 1900, p. 44.)

VOGL, A. (1950). The discovery of the organic mercurial diuretics. *American Heart Journal*, **39**, 881-883.

WILDER, R. M. (1921). The effect of ketonemia on the course of epilepsy. *Mayo Clinic Bulletin*, **2**, No. 307.

Observation, Hypothesis, Experimentation: II

I want to consider now the preliminaries to the development of a hypothesis, what I have referred to previously as ' observation '. In fact, research does not have to depend upon inspired observations. The questions which we hope will be answered by appropriate research are there facing us all the time. The experienced research worker is acutely aware of the innumerable problems which face him and from which he has to make a selection in order to get down to specific activity. In contrast to this, the most difficult problem that faces a beginner in research is that of finding a problem, i.e. finding the sort of hypothesis which gives him a question which can be answered by investigation. The difference between the beginner and the experienced man is very much a question of attitude. The training of a medical undergraduate takes a long time, not only because he requires this time in order to develop the necessary skill to practice medicine but also because he has to acquire a large amount of background information on which his skill is based. In consequence, he tends to accept his teaching uncritically. He does so because his interest is concerned predominantly with the problems of learning how to manage sick people. The research worker has exactly the opposite kind of attitude. He doubts everything, and when one starts to do this it is astonishing how insecure are the foundations of the practice of medicine. Every so often I have an experience which is common to all psychiatrists: my medical and surgical colleagues commiserate with me on the fact that I practice in a branch of medicine which, they believe, is lacking in background information. My reply to this is to issue them with a challenge. I undertake to open any standard textbook of medicine or surgery at random and I am prepared to bet them that on the two pages thus exposed I will find at least one statement which is blatantly untrue and another one for which no evidence is available. I have not yet had any acceptance of this challenge! Of course, this is not the fault of the writers of textbooks. Medicine is an ancient craft and much of the knowledge on which it is based is of old and of traditional origin. Many of our accepted beliefs have never been tested by the scientific method and even for those that have some evidence backing them, that evidence would be regarded as inadequate nowadays. In any case, the problems that we have to deal with now are very different from those in the past, and often the facts and information which was appropriate then is not so now.

So, when young doctors come to me and ask for advice and help in organizing a research project, say for an M.D., the first thing they ask me is how to make a start, how to find a problem. My advice is invariably to say, ' Look at your work and consider the problems that face you, especially the common ones. Ask yourself " what information do I need in order to be able to solve these problems?" ' Although I am talking about clinical medicine and in terms of clinical research, this way of looking at one's problems applies just as much to those branches of medicine which are relatively remote from the clinic, such as bacteriology or pathology. It applies also to all those professions associated with medicine, such as social workers, psychologists and so on. Even then it is necessary to have an intimate knowledge of the field against which the particular problem must be seen.

Knowledge of Background

In general, there are three ways in which one can find out what is known about the subject, how things stand. The first one is by reading, the second is by experience and the third is by information from others. The first is the least reliable, the second is the best, the third is easiest.

You already have some notion why the first is the least reliable. You all know how difficult it is to judge the value of what you read until you already have some experience in the field and know exactly what is going on. Sometimes, of course, you can tell by just looking at the name of the author! The reason why I always recommend young doctors to attend conferences and congresses as often as they can is that they get an opportunity to meet the people who write the articles and books which they have on their reading list. It has been said that this is the quickest way of shortening the list, but it does work the other way too! Reading requires judgement, which is very difficult to acquire, but there is no substitute for reading.

Incidentally, when you read up some subject, go to the original papers for evaluating the results. Time and again you will find, when you go to the original papers, that the authors who did the work expressed certain qualifications and doubts about the findings they had made. The reviewers, the summarizers and the writers of textbooks who copy from them tend to drop out the qualifications and doubts, and the material becomes more and more assured and categorical. I mention one actual example: for many years it used to be said that when the sympathetic nerves were stimulated, their effect was due to the release of adrenalin from the nerve-endings. When one looked at the original papers it turned out that the effect of sympathetic stimulation was not quite like adrenalin, and so the original workers had postulated a substance which they called ' Sympathin ', because it came from the sympathetic nerves. They said that it obviously was very like adrenalin and probably could be, but there were some slight differences between them. Further experiments showed that their doubts were well founded and it became necessary to postulate the two ' sympathins ', sympathin E and sympathin I.

Since the end of the War, it has been shown that the original provisos were justified, because the effect of sympathetic stimulation is not the simulation of adrenalin, but, in many cases, more like the simulation of noradrenalin. In nature, these two substances are secreted in different proportions and since they have different effects, it is not surprising that the sympathetic nervous system does not reproduce exactly the effect of the injection of a pure substance. I must warn you that even the simple statements I have just made are subject to qualification. The last word on the subject has not by any means been said. Incidentally, it is a point to remember, when writing up your own work, to be cautious about it, for your own sake. Modesty never does any harm, particularly if some one comes along and shows that your findings are nonsense!

The second way to acquire knowledge of the background is by experience. Unfortunately, it takes many, many years and even then is always limited. Finally, learning from others is clearly the easiest way of obtaining what one wants. On this point you may remember that old saying that second best to knowing something yourself, if not as good or even better, is knowing whom to ask, knowing somebody who does know it. Even if you do not get the information you want, you may learn where to find it. This brings up the advantages of starting research with collaborators. If you work in a research unit, your colleagues are more or less acquainted with other people in the same field, they are aware of the difficulties, they know about the problems that arise, they know what has been done and what has not been done. If you go into such a unit, willing to learn, prepared to accept instructions and advice, you will be given a job which is not too difficult to start off with. You will learn how to straighten out difficulties and gradually you will begin to get the feel of this particular type of work.

I must remind you once again, that if you want to plan some research or do an investigation in the clinical field, you have to consult a clinician, for only he has that necessary experience.

Hypothesis

Before starting on the formulation of the hypothesis I want to give some definitions so that you will be quite clear what I am talking about. The word ' treatment ' is used to mean any procedure which the experimenter uses on his subjects. In clinical medicine it will be used to signify drugs or hormones, physical treatments such as gamma-ray radiation for the treatment of cancer and short-wave diathermy in physiotherapeutics. It would also be applied to a training method for rehabilitation of injured limbs. In surgery, the term applies obviously to surgical procedures but could include such additions as preliminary blood transfusions or saline infusions and so on. ' Treatment ' can also be used to apply to many other active procedures, e.g. a stimulus applied to a peripheral nerve in order to measure rate of conduction will also count as a treatment. When a social worker wants to compare the sort of information she obtains when she interviews a patient in the clinic or at home then these two locations for the interview can be regarded as different ' treatments '. The same will apply when she wants to compare the effects of interviewing the patient in the presence or absence of the spouse. If I want to evaluate different methods of teaching medical students, then these different methods will be called treatments.

The ' subject ' is the recipient of the treatment. As a clinician, I tend to apply the term ' patient ' to a sick person and ' subject ' to a healthy one, but when I am talking about the design of an experiment they are both subjects. A subject need not necessarily be a single individual. For example, if I were investigating the effects of different treatments for marital problems, the ' subject ' would be a married couple.

A ' factor ' classifies the subjects into at least two groups. The factor sex will have two groups, male and female; the factor marital status will include single, married, divorced, widowed, etc. A continuous variable such as age or blood pressure can be used as a factor if it is divided into a set of groups which are mutually exclusive. Finally, treatment itself can be regarded as a factor, when we compare two or more treatments. It is implicit that the different subgroups or ' levels ' of a factor have different effects on the results of treatment and the experiment will provide evidence whether this is so.

Once you have found your general problem, it is then necessary to clarify it and define it. In this way you break it down into a number of separate parts each of which gives you a hypothesis which is the basis of an experiment. Each one of these parts is a unit hypothesis which determines a unit experiment.

Of course you do not have to do only one experiment, one unit at a time. You can do many simultaneously, but you will not get any information that is definite and you will not have an adequate basis for making inferences until you have broken down your general problem into its units. Then you can answer each unit with the appropriate experiment. Perhaps that is put too forcibly, but I want to emphasize the value of such a procedure in making clear your problems and the answers.

DEFINITION OF HYPOTHESIS

Suppose I have a new tranquillizer which looks as if it might be useful for treating mental patients. Such a statement is too vague. Does ' mental illness ' mean schizophrenias, depressions, etc., or all diagnoses? By ' patients ' do I mean those acutely ill or chronically ill? I can decide what I like but I must make some sort of decision. I can classify patients any way I want to : on the basis of diagnostic categories or of psychodynamics, but I must make the decision and say what sort of patients I mean. Either the drug is useful for every patient or only to some, and if the latter, I must say which. Again and again one sees this essential criterion forgotten.

Having defined the kind of patient, I must now consider what I mean by drug. Since the drug is already named I must now define the dose. There is little value in administering insufficient treatment and a trial which showed that a drug was ineffective may have done so simply because the drug was given in too small a dose. The correct dose may have to be determined by some preliminary experiments. After all, one gives atropine in fractions of milligrams; one gives aspirin in fractions of a gram and more. Having decided on the dose to be given I must then decide on the method of administration; there is not much use in giving small doses of penicillin by mouth although large ones are effective. It is useless to give a treatment the wrong way. A definition of treatment therefore includes the description of an adequate quantity given in a particular way to produce the desired effect. But how long does it take? Will the effect appear in minutes, hours, days, weeks, months or years? That too must be stated.

Then I have to say what I mean by improvement. This is one of the most difficult of problems. I am reminded of the story of the patient who used to suffer from hay fever. A friend of his met him one day and asked how he was getting on. 'How's the hay fever?' 'Oh, that's gone, I don't suffer from it any more'. His friend asks, 'How did you do it?' 'Oh, I have injections every week from January to June'. 'I see', said his friend 'you now suffer from injections'. In dealing with diabetes mellitus one is faced with the problem that the diabetic who suffers from certain symptoms and who is then put on a diet with injections, finds that he has merely exchanged one misfortune for another. It is true that he doesn't feel weak and he doesn't feel thirsty; now he feels perpetually hungry and he is continually being pricked. He cannot go out because he cannot eat food outside and he cannot mix with his friends because they all look at him and stare when he starts to measure his food and calculate his calories. It is not therefore surprising that those who have practical experience in the treatment of diabetes are not so impressed with the value of insulin injections, the scales of diets, the tables of calories and so on. They find that if too much emphasis is placed on these things, many patients just give up and decide that they would rather enjoy what is left of their life than drag out the rest in misery. So one has to remember that 'improvement' is not quite such a simple matter as might appear at first sight. The patient who suffers from duodenal ulcer and who is cured of it by the surgeon who removes his stomach, is not very happy when he now finds he suffers from dumping syndrome. Is a patient improved when he exchanges the symptoms of hypertension for those of postural hypotension? I give these examples because it is sometimes thought that only in psychiatry is there difficulty in deciding what is meant by improvement. In all branches of medicine, improvement is a very difficult matter to be clear about, and what is meant by it must be decided beforehand.

Now this process of specifying the details of a particular question comes down to defining a particular unit experiment. If you say that the drug will be given in a particular dose, then that is one experiment, and the conclusions you draw from it are not necessarily applicable to treatment given with another dose. If you try the treatment on a specified group of patients then you cannot conclude that another group of patients, of a different kind, will respond in the same way. The conclusion from the experiment may apply to them, or it may not. You cannot be certain. If you want to know whether it does apply to another group of patients then you must include that group in your experiment; or rather, you must now have two experiments each dealing with a separate group of patients. This gives you two unit experiments. You can do them simultaneously, but your two groups of patients must be clearly distinguished in your work. This then is the process of developing your hypothesis; you clarify and define your various generalizations until each one is made into a specific statement. Then each specific statement is the basis for a specific experiment and that is your unit experiment.

As I pointed out in the last lecture, the evaluation of a treatment always requires some standard for comparison. The most obvious standard is that based on previous experience, but this can be very unsatisfactory. It takes a long time to get this experience and if you have to wait several years before you can start an experiment, then advance is going to be very slow. Even more important than this is the fact that past experience can give rise to false results because of constant changes that have occurred over the course of time. Consider the case of a psychotherapist. As he goes on, his experience increases and therefore his ability increases, but other changes occur as well, he grows older and this may give rise to increasing prestige with his patients; patients are likely to respect an older psychotherapist more than a young or youthful-looking one. This may play a part in his effectiveness. A surgeon's skill may also increase with the passing of the years.

Other difficulties may arise. We may develop new diagnostic methods for detecting disorders and, consequently, the type of case which goes under the same name as before becomes changed. The case of general paresis is a good example. Once we start routine analysis of the contents of spinal fluid, we can detect the disorder in its very early stages long before it can be detected clinically. The result is that the classical type of general paresis is now relatively uncommon. Other factors play their part. In mental disorder the facilities available for treatment themselves affect the type of case seen. The introduction of voluntary admission to a mental hospital results in a milder type of patient being admitted. As soon as the process for discharge and readmission of patients becomes simple and flexible, the average length of stay in hospital immediately tends to diminish; but at the same time the number of readmissions increases. A simple change, of law or of regulations, can therefore completely destroy the relevance of former experience in relation to the present.

Furthermore, we have a phenomenon which is not often recognized, a secular change in the nature of the disease itself. Scarlatina was a dangerous, killing disease in the latter part of the nineteenth century. It is now, a very minor, almost a trivial one. In my own field of work, there is a very well known example of such change. The classical hysterias, described in the late nineties by Charcot, Janet and Freud just do not appear nowadays. You can find them if you look hard enough but they are extremely rare. It is unlikely, however, that hysteria has disappeared, it has changed its form.

The simplest type of experiment that gives the comparison we need is the type known as before-and-after. For example we can investigate the effects of exercise on the circulation and we make our observations on the circulation before and after the exercise. We can make the experiment more complicated and investigate another factor by carrying it out under conditions where the subject breathes air with different proportions of oxygen. We could start by investigating the effects on the circulation when he is breathing air which contains 20 per cent oxygen and then we could give him artificial airs containing 30, 40, 50 up to 100 per cent of oxygen. In each case we examine the circulation at rest and then after exercise during the appropriate conditions. Unfortunately, this sort of experiment is rarely possible. If we try to compare the effects of different antibiotics for the treatment of, say, enteric fever, we cannot investigate the individual while he is well and then give him the antibiotic when he falls ill in order to measure his return to health. We can take a number of sick patients and give them one antibiotic and estimate the recovery. We cannot then go on to give a second antibiotic to those patients who have recovered. To make this sort of comparison we have to take two groups of patients, and give each group one of the two antibiotics. On this basis we can now start to make comparisons but it is obvious that there are many difficulties involved in this, and these are the problems we shall consider in the technique of experimentation. Incidentally, one of the problems of doing repeated experiments on one subject is that the information obtained applies only to that one individual. Extension to other persons cannot be guaranteed. Hence the need for replication on more than one subject.

A Simple Experiment

Let us consider the data obtained from a hypothetical experiment. This would consist of two treatments applied to five subjects each and the results measured in some sort of way. If to specify the experiment would make you feel happier I would suggest that we could assume that the experiment consisted of two kinds of visual stimulus applied to the subjects and the criterion consists of the changes in the EEG; it could be two kinds of hypoglycaemic or hypotensive drug, the criterion being the drop in blood sugar or blood pressure. We could use two different treatments given to patients suffering from rheumatoid arthritis or depressive illness and measure their improvement by means of a rating scale. For your convenience, the actual measurements have been converted into index numbers which are all small integers.

The results are as follows:

Group 1   3, 5, 8, 10, 12   Total 38
Group 2   1, 4, 6, 7, 13   Total 31

It is obvious that group 2 has done less well than group 1, for its total, and average score, is less. Careful examination shows that each subject has a different score from the others, whether within the same group or in both groups. Furthermore, the highest score in group 2 is greater than the highest score in group 1; at the same time, the lowest score in group 2 is lower than the lowest score in group 1. The great differences between individual subjects must make us wary about drawing conclusions on the differences between treatments. We do not know if the treatments differ in their effects. The differences that we get between the two groups could be due entirely to the differences between individuals. Since we did not know how the individuals would respond to the treatments before the experiment, then the differences between the two treatments might be due entirely to chance, the way the patients were selected for each treatment. We therefore have two interpretations of the results of this experiment. The first is that the difference between the two groups is due to the treatments, and the second is that the difference is entirely due to chance. The second one is known as the ' null hypothesis '. We have to find some way of distinguishing between the effects of the treatments and the effects of chance and this requires the use of some form of statistical analysis.

Applicability of Statistics

Even nowadays, we can still find clinicians who believe that statistics cannot be applied to the clinical field. They argue that every patient is unique and therefore statistics cannot be applied to clinical problems. This argument is standing on its head: statistics are applicable precisely because every patient is unique. If all patients were alike, or those in one category were exactly alike, you would never do anything more than to try a treatment on one, and you would know the answer for all. It is because of the variability that occurs, because every person is unique, that statistical methods must be used.

Suppose I want to do a fixing job in my home, using nuts and bolts. I go to my cupboard to fetch them and find, to my astonishment, that I have only bolts and cannot find any nuts. I take one of the bolts and go to the local hardware stores and show it to the salesman. He tests the bolt on different sizes of nuts and finds one that matches. Thereupon I buy a packet of this size of nuts from him. You notice that only one bolt was used and only one nut was found to be satisfactory; thereupon I buy a whole packet and I know that when I return home all the nuts will fit all the bolts. The reason is that all the bolts are the same size and all the nuts also, so if one bolt fits a nut then all will fit all of them. It is because they are all identical (within the limits required) that it is sufficient to test only one and know that the results of the test apply to all.

Summary

The practice of medicine is still based on very limited knowledge and problems face us in every aspect of our practical work. We have to examine the literature on the subject to help us clarify these problems. In order to carry out research on these problems, we have to define them very specifically and in this way form hypotheses which can be tested by experimental investigation. We have to define clearly the treatment, the subjects and the criterion which will measure the effect of the treatment. To evaluate the effect of a treatment we must have knowledge of a background state. Since the subjects differ among themselves, we cannot absolutely distinguish the effects of treatment from chance results and the latter form the basis of the null hypothesis. Because subjects differ it is necessary to use statistical methods to draw conclusions.

REFERENCE

BROWNING, J. S. & HOUSEWORTH, J. H. (1953). Development of new symptoms following medical and surgical treatment for duodenal ulcer. *Psychosomatic Medicine*, **15**, 328-336.

Induction: II

STATISTICS ARE NOT EVERYTHING

In the last lecture I referred briefly to an (hypothetical) experiment but refrained from considering the problems related to experimentation. The reason for this is that although a good experiment rests upon a proper formulation of its hypothesis, is must be so designed that valid conclusions can be drawn from it. Beginners find this the most difficult aspect of research and I shall therefore consider this now.

The drawing of conclusions from a clinical investigation is generally done in statistical terms. Clinical medicine is at a stage when the average clinician still tends to feel that this is an unnecessary intrusion. Why should the statistician have to come into clinical medicine? Many of the greatest achievements in this field have been done without the benefit of statistics; one could even say ' most of them ' without being far wrong. The traditional methods of observation, clinical judgement and experience have served medicine very well, and there is surely no reason to assume that they will not do so in the future. This attitude is reinforced by the fact that the application of modern experimental methods, supplemented by statistical analysis, has tended to be very iconoclastic: traditional methods of treatment have been subjected to elaborate testing, and after some complicated juggling of figures, have been found wanting. The clinician is beginning to feel harried! Every time he prescribes a treatment he feels that the statistician is peering over his shoulder and criticizing his efforts.

Of course, great progress has been made in medicine without the use of statistical analysis, and it will continue. Let us take a simple example to illustrate the point. I quote from a paper on ' Laboratory diagnosis of galactosaemia at birth ':

Normal blood : $3 \cdot 5$ μg galactose/ml red cells (mean)

$0 \cdot 7$–$9 \cdot 8$ μg galactose/ml red cells (range)

Galactosaemic blood : Case 1 : 58 μg/ml

Case 2 : 76 μg/ml.

It is obvious that statistics are not required to demonstrate the difference between normal and galactosaemic blood.

When we are investigating great differences between groups, or grossly pathological phenomena, we do not need refined statistical methods to demonstrate them. When Addison and Bright were observing the diseases which have been named after them, they needed nothing more than the careful observation of a few cases to prove their point. The value of liver for the treatment of Addison's anaemia, or of insulin for diabetes mellitus, can be demonstrated on a few patients, without any statistical analysis of the results. These are gross phenomena, and that makes the problem easy. I have no doubt that the future developments will yield plenty of such examples, but most of the progress of clinical medicine depends on the continued investigation of relatively minor changes. To elucidate these we need the best of techniques and these include statistical methods.

Correlation and Causation

In any case statistical inferences are not the only ones which are based on data. A fallacy which is very prevalent in ordinary thinking (particularly political!) but is quite common in our field, concerns the difference between correlation and causation. 'If one thing goes with another then it must have caused it.' I once read in the medical press a number of years ago, a statement which pointed out that all through the twentieth century cancer had been increasing and that this was exactly paralleled by the increase in the use of aluminium cooking vessels. In the writer's opinion, the cause of cancer was the aluminium which was coming into the food. That may sound silly to us now, but it was not quite so silly in the '20s or '30s, and I assure you and I hope you will believe me, that I will be able to find just such off-beat notions as this at the present time.

I once saw a paper which pointed out that appendicitis had suddenly appeared round about the end of the nineteenth century and then became increasingly prevalent. It pointed out that this occurred parallel with the sudden increase in the consumption of sugar, denatured sugar, and it was argued that the two were related. The author then proposed the plausible notion that excessive sugar in the diet produced a different kind of fermentation in the intestines, it alters the flora of the intestines, favouring the development of pathogenic varieties, and this produced appendicitis. It is a good story indeed and very plausible; as good a story as anyone hears about schizophrenia or psoriasis.

Another example, one that is of great importance nowadays, is the increasing occurrence of coronary thrombosis. As you know, it has been shown that this is correlated with an increase in the consumption of fats. This has been demonstrated in many different countries and for a number of years. This is an important fact but its meaning is a matter for experimental determination. After all, it has been pointed out that the incidence of coronary thrombosis has increased quite steadily and correspondingly with the increase in the number of radios. Now, there is a great difference between the hypothesis that the increase in coronary thrombosis is due to the increased consumption of fat, and the hypothesis that it is due to the increased number of radio sets sold. The difference is the presence of a theory. There is a good theory to explain the former, and none to explain the latter. I admit there was a theory to account for the relation between appendicitis and the consumption of sugar. A good theory is very important, but it is only a beginning. In the end we will have to experiment, and it is the results of experiments that are the final arbiters that one must accept. As Roger Bacon put it, ' Neither the voice of authority, nor the weight of reason and argument are as significant as experiment, for thence comes quiet to the mind '.

A DIFFICULT INFERENCE

I would like to give you an example of drawing conclusions from figures which differs considerably from the sort of problems I shall be considering in due course. It is related to the problems of correlation that I have just mentioned, and illustrates the fallacies that lie in wait when one wishes to make a prediction from data pertaining to the past. The material is taken from an investigation on the relation between epilepsy and convulsions in infancy. It was found that of the epileptics attending hospital, 34 per cent had a history of attacks of convulsions in the first two years of life. A control series had only 2 per cent of individuals with such a history. Among epileptics 34 per cent or one in three, and only 2 per cent or one in fifty, in the others. It was therefore concluded that convulsions in the first two years of life were to be taken as a manifestation of epilepsy and on this basis it was recommended that if children had convulsions within the first two years of life they should be given anti-epileptic treatment in the hope of averting the disorder.

This sounds very plausible until one thinks about it. What is the incidence of epilepsy in the population as a whole? It is about 1 per cent. Now let us consider a population of 10,000 persons. They will have one hundred epileptics among them, and consequently there will be 9900 who will not have epilepsy. Of the hundred epileptics, according to the findings, 34 will have had a history of convulsions and therefore 66 will not have had such a history. Of the 9900 non-epileptics, two in a hundred will have had a history of convulsions, i.e. 198, and the rest will not have had such a history. It will be clearer if we put it in the form of a table.

TABLE 4.1

	With convulsions	Without convulsions	Total
Epileptics	34	66	100
Non-epileptics	198	9702	9900
TOTAL	232	9768	10000

Let us now look at the children who have convulsions: There are 232 in this population of 10,000, and 34 subsequently developed epilepsy, which is a ratio of one in seven. There are 9768 who do not have convulsions and 66 subsequently develop epilepsy, a ratio of one in 148. So, to have convulsions in infancy means that the chance of developing epilepsy is increased from one in 148 to one in seven, a very great increase. There is no doubt that convulsions in infancy are related to the development of epilepsy in adult life; but remember this, of those who have had convulsions only one in seven develop epilepsy, so six do not. There is still six to one chance against the development of epilepsy in a child who has had convulsions. It would be absurd to suggest that seven children should be given anti-epileptic drugs for many, many years in the hope that one might not develop epilepsy.

This point is a very important one. We meet it again and again, and although I deliberately chose an example from general medicine, it is all too prevalent in the field of psychiatry. Consider schizophrenia for example. Let us take the exaggerated notion that every schizophrenic has had a schizoid personality or showed a schizoid type of behaviour before falling ill. Does this mean that persons who show schizoid behaviour in childhood or adolescence are going to develop schizophrenia or, at least, more likely than not? Not in the least bit! This is so even if every schizophrenic had such a history, without exception, and we know that this is not the case.

Let us return to the problems of infantile convulsions and epilepsy. If you look at the following invented table, you will see that the original arguments are quite true: children who had convulsions would overwhelmingly tend to develop epilepsy in adult life. Out of 36 children with convulsions 34 would become epileptic.

TABLE 4.2

	With infantile convulsions	Without infantile convulsions	Total
Epileptics	34	66	100
Non-epileptics	2	98	100
TOTAL	36	164	200

This is an unrealistic table, for you will see that the incidence of epilepsy is 50 per cent of the population. The next table marks the dividing line:

TABLE 4.3

	With infantile convulsions	Without infantile convulsions	Total
Epileptics	34	66	100
Non-epileptics	34	1666	1700
TOTAL	68	1732	1800

With the same basic proportions of 34 per cent and 2 per cent, it can be seen that there is now an even chance that a child who has convulsions will subsequently develop epilepsy. This occurs when the rate of epilepsy in the population is 100 in 1800, or 5·6 per cent. Were the incidence of epilepsy to be above this rate, convulsions in infancy would indicate a more than even chance of developing epilepsy. An incidence below 5·6 per cent would lead to the reverse inference, even though the figures of 34 per cent and 2 per cent are unchanged.

I hope I have not confused you with so many tables and figures.

Let us look at the problem without figures. The original argument based on the data was concerned with probabilities, i.e. the chances that a child who has an attack of convulsions will develop epilepsy later on in life. I have shown you that the estimate of these probabilities can vary from very small to very large, depending on the conditions. The correct estimate can only be made by taking into account one aspect of the problem of drawing conclusions from a sample about the whole population.

If, as Freud stated over half a century ago, all neurotics have a history of an unresolved Oedipus complex, is it true that an unresolved Oedipus complex will always produce neurosis? Obviously not. It is quite true that many neurotics have had a bad childhood; many, but not all. If it comes to that, there is scarcely one of us whose parents have not broken some, if not most, of the rules for bringing up children, according to the books that give advice on that subject. In spite of that we have come through without much harm; we have friends (and enemies), we have jobs and pay our taxes.

The fact that particular characteristics can be found in patients does not prove that they are the causes of their disorder. That is to say, they may be necessary, but they may not be sufficient. This is obvious enough when we are dealing with such well established phenomena as infection with diphtheria or tubercle bacilli. In the field of psychiatry, and especially of the neuroses, we do not know of any factor which is necessary. Remember, these problems are not questions of figures or statistics, even though they may appear in that form. They concern the drawing of conclusions from the evidence, a matter of logic, or if you like plain common sense. Nevertheless, you will find this sort of fallacy in the literature only too often.

The Null Hypothesis

Let us return to the simple ' experiment ' that I described in the previous lecture. You will remember that I pointed out that, since we do not know whether the two treatments differ, but we do know that the subjects differ, it is conceivable that the differences between the two groups were not due to the differences between the treatments but between the subjects. This alternative explanation is known as the *null hypothesis*. Until you have grasped this notion, you will not understand the principles of experimentation and how to draw conclusions from data.

It is always possible that the difference between treatments which we have obtained is due to chance, i.e. the way the individual subjects were selected, and therefore we can never disprove the null hypothesis. What we can do is to design experiments in such a way as to make the null hypothesis as unlikely as possible. We have also to determine how unlikely, or likely, it is, otherwise we cannot tell what the results signify. If we know that the probability of the null hypothesis is small then we can safely reject it. We can assert that we believe that the results are not due to chance but are due to the differences between treatments, and we can be reasonably assured of our belief.

Two Types of Error

Of course, we cannot be absolutely certain. A rare event will occur with its own particular frequency, as Fisher pointed out, and it will do so however surprising it may be that it should occur to us. When we refuse to accept the null hypothesis we may be wrong and this incorrect rejection of the null hypothesis is known as type 1 error. Let me try to make this clearer. In our experiment we found that there was a difference between treatments and if, therefore, we reject the null hypothesis although there really is no difference between them, then we are, in the jargon of horse racing, backing a loser. That is type 1 error.

The reverse of this is type 2 error. It is the incorrect acceptance of the null hypothesis, or if you like, missing a winner. The experiment showed a difference but it may be small compared to the effects of chance factors. We therefore decide that it is probably a chance result and accept the null hypothesis, that the difference between the two treatments is due to chance when in fact it is not, and so we ' miss a winner '.

We can never completely eliminate these two kinds of error but we can design our experiment to reduce them to a minimum. We have to design it in such a way that it can demonstrate differences, when they exist, and we do this by making the probability of the null hypothesis as low as possible. You will now see why Fisher said (and I abbreviate the quotation a little) ' every experiment exists to disprove the null hypothesis ', although at first sight this may seem an extraordinarily odd way of looking at the nature of experimentation.

EXPERIMENTAL ' PROOF '

The usual way of looking at experiments is to regard them as proving a positive rather than disproving a negative. This is mistaken. When an experiment is done to test a theory, its results can only conform with that theory, not prove it; for it is always possible to devise other theories that will be equally satisfied by the experimental results. This is not mere speculation, for the history of science is full of examples of theories which have been used to explain empirical facts and which have subsequently been replaced by other theories, explaining the same facts (but, of course, additional ones too). Even when we consider the simplest type of experiment, designed to test the value of a particular treatment, it is extremely unwise to assume that we have proved what we intended to. The results of a treatment may be due to an unknown or inconspicuous part of the treatment we give. An example of this is the way that copper and manganese were found to be essential in the treatment of iron-deficiency anaemias. It took a long time to clarify what aspects of rehabilitation after fractures were the important ones, and we still do not know the essential factors of social treatment of chronic schizophrenics or of psychotherapy.

It is also impossible to prove the null hypothesis; for example, you cannot prove that two treatments are equally good, that one is no better than the other. Even if you do not find any difference between them, it may be that you have not taken enough cases to demonstrate the slight difference that does exist. Had you gone on long enough you would have found the difference; and you can always go on longer. It might be argued that such minute differences are of no interest anyway, that one is looking for a reasonable difference. In that case, you have to decide beforehand what you would call a reasonable difference, and as you will see later, that brings you back to very much the same situation.

Probability of the Null Hypothesis

How do we determine the probability of the null hypothesis? Let us first be quite clear what it is. It states that the difference obtained between the two groups could have been due to the differences between the persons. We had originally ten subjects and we selected five for one treatment and the other five for the other treatment. Assuming the null hypothesis to be true, we have first to determine what every possible result could have been with these ten cases. Had we selected them differently we would have obtained different results. We might have obtained this: group 1: 3, 5, 10, 12, 13, Total 43, and group 2: 1, 4, 6, 7, 8, Total 26, which would have shown an even greater effect for the treatment of group 1; but then we might have had this: group 1: 3, 4, 5, 7, 10. Total 29, and group 2: 1, 6, 8, 12, 13, Total 40, which would have shown a greater effect for group 2!

We have to select five subjects out of ten to form one group and there are 252 ways of doing this so that no group contains exactly the same subjects as the others. Those of you who remember your combinatorial theory from your school days will know how this is calculated, and those who do not will have to take my word for it. Now, although the subjects in any one of these 252 groups differ from those in the others, the total scores of many of the groups are the same. We now construct a table showing how many of the groups obtained a given score. If you prefer it, you can divide the total by five and show the mean score.

TABLE 4.4.   *Frequency distribution of total scores in group 1*

Score	Frequency	Cumulative frequency (descending)	Cumulative frequency (ascending)	Score	Frequency	Cumulative frequency (descending)	Cumulative frequency (ascending)
19	1	1	252	35	16	142	126
20	1	2	251	36	14	156	110
21	2	4	250	37	15	171	96
22	2	6	248	38	13	184	81
23	4	10	246	39	13	197	68
24	3	13	242	40	11	208	55
25	6	19	239	41	10	218	44
26	7	26	233	42	8	226	34
27	8	34	226	43	7	233	26
28	10	44	218	44	6	239	19
29	11	55	208	45	3	242	13
30	13	68	197	46	4	246	10
31	13	81	184	47	2	248	6
32	15	96	171	48	2	250	4
33	14	110	156	49	1	251	2
34	16	126	142	50	1	252	1

In whatever way we select the subjects to make the two groups, the total number of subjects is the same ten. Group 2 had a total score of 31 points and group 1 38 points. The total score for the two groups is therefore 69, and the difference between the scores of the two groups was seven points. Since we did the experiment in order to look for differences, a difference of more than seven points would have been even more convincing. In other words, if group 2 had had a total score of 30 points or 29 or less, then group 1 would have a score of 39, 40 or more. If we look at the table, we see that there are 13 of the groups who would have had a score of 31 and if we take all those who had a total score of 31 or less the number of such groups is 81. Now, when we carried out the experiment we were looking for differences between the treatments; we had no reason to believe that one treatment was better than the other, all that concerned us was the difference between them. It would have been just as meaningful therefore had group 2 had a score of 38 and group 1 of 31 and if you look at the table you will see that 81 of such groups would have had a score of 38 and upwards in group 2 or, if you prefer it, 31 and less in group 1. Out of 252 ways of selecting the two groups of subjects, 162 would therefore have shown a difference of seven points or more between the two groups. The probability of getting such a result is therefore $162/252 = \cdot643$. More clearly, out of the 252 possible ways of selecting two groups of subjects from the ten, 64·3 per cent would have shown a difference of seven points or more in their total score. It is therefore more likely than not that the results could be due to chance and therefore we must accept the null hypothesis. In other words, the data do not provide any evidence to suggest that the treatments differ.*

This way of determining the probability of the null hypothesis or, in statistical language, testing for statistical significance, is simple and absolute in the sense that it involves no presuppositions whatsoever. This is the Randomization test. It is rarely used in practice because it is too laborious. There are 252 ways of splitting ten subjects into equal groups, to split 14 subjects will give 3,432 ways, 16 subjects give 12,870 and 18 give 48,620. This is too many even for modern computers.

I want to make one final point. We could not reject the null hypothesis because it had a probability of 0·63. We would have done the same had it been 0·5. Had the probability been 0·4, 0·3 or 0·2 we would have been less and less sure about rejecting it. At what point do we decide that the probability of the null hypothesis is so low that we are safe in rejecting it? When the probability P is as low as 0·05, it is assumed that we are fairly safe in rejecting the null hypothesis and we therefore state that the differences between the treatments is ' significant '. If P is 0·01 or less we say the differences are

---

* I am indebted to Professor Ardie Lubin for this way of introducing tests of significance.

very significant and if P is less than 0·001 we say that they are highly significant. If we use a level of significance of 0·05 it means that, in the long run, out of 100 experiments we do we shall be wrong, in rejecting the null hypothesis, five times. Making a fool of yourself five times out of 100 investigations is therefore what I mean when I say that you are ' safe '!

Strictly speaking, you should decide, before you carry out the experiment, what level of significance you would consider appropriate. This will depend very much on the background of information that you have about the experiment and what is involved in accepting the experiment as successful. The problem of designing clinical experiments and drawing conclusions from them are logical or statistical, but when it comes to taking action on them, the problems are clinical. They may also be quite practical ones such as difficulty, expense, and so on. Suppose a clinician tests a new treatment and he finds that either the new treatment is better than the old, or that there is a 7 per cent probability that his ' improvement ' is a chance result. Then if the new treatment is simple, easy, or no more expensive than the old, it might be well to adopt it. However, if it were difficult, required much training to use, needed a large staff, or were very expensive, the decision might then be that the evidence in favour of the new treatment was insufficient to warrant going to all that trouble and expense. The conclusion from the experiment is determined by the result: it could have been due to chance in seven out of a hundred times. Practical action based on the results is determined by all sorts of other factors. One form of practical action would be to decide to continue the experiment in order to obtain more convincing evidence, i.e. to get a result which could have appeared by chance only one in a hundred or one in a thousand times.

Summary

Statistical methods of inference are necessary when the effects of treatments are not large in comparison with the effects of chance. The null hypothesis is always possible and we design our experiments to make it as improbable as we can. We can then safely reject it although we may still be in error. The probability of the null hypothesis is the ' significance ' and a simple hypothetical experiment demonstrated how this could be calculated.

REFERENCES

SCHWARTZ, V., HOLZEL, A. & KOMROWER, E. M. (1958). Laboratory diagnosis of congenital galactosaemia at birth. *Lancet*, **i**, 24-25.

Observation, Hypothesis: III

If there are no particular observations which have aroused your curiosity, there are two ways of finding a project of research. The first is to look at your problems; but, as I have already mentioned, the beginner is apt to think of his problems in far too general terms. We do not do research on rheumatoid arthritis, schizophrenia or cancer; but what we can do, for example, is to look at the differences between those patients who respond to a particular treatment and those who do not. If it is known that patients suffering from a particular disorder sometimes show a given biochemical change, then we could ask ourselves what is the difference between the clinical manifestations of the illness in those patients who show the change and those who do not. If you look through the literature on the subject it is extremely likely that you will find some clue or suggestion of lead as to where you go from there. The second way is to doubt accepted 'truths', and the more obvious they are the greater the need to question them. Retarded depression, it is said, is associated with early morning wakening; women suffering from gall bladder disease are 'fair fat and forty'. Are you really sure? The literature on the subject should give you the answer to your questions but it is very rare indeed that it does. The initial step having been made, the rest is simple though laborious. You must look up the literature, in the first case to find out what has been done about your particular problem and in the second, to see what is the evidence backing these traditional beliefs.

Search of the Literature

The medical curriculum is already so full that it is not surprising that students are not taught how to search the literature. I do not think that this is all important or that very much should be done about it, because I believe that the medical curriculum should be shortened rather than lengthened. To postgraduates, knowing how to search the literature is a basic skill and that is why I am going to talk about it now. There are plenty of books on the subject but they are rather forbidding as they tend to work on the assumption that the search of the literature is intended to cover all of it. If you are going to write a review of progress on a subject, or to give an account of its history, or try to produce a complete bibliography for some particular purpose, then these books are essential reading. If you are going to search the literature merely as the preliminary to planning a project, then the procedure is really very much simpler.

The most obvious way is to start by looking at those text books, usually of the more comprehensive kind, which give references. It is true that these may be out of date, but that does not matter, as you can always fill in the gaps up to the most recent work. Unfortunately, text-books tend to gloss over difficulties and problems and in trying to give a clear account of the state of the knowledge, ignore the doubt and difficulties. In this respect, you will find that monographs are much more helpful, but you must know which ones to look at and here the text books will give you some guidance. For more recent work, the best procedure is to look at the annual reviews in your particular subject as these are very convenient of access. You can supplement this by looking at the index of the last year or two in your favourite journal. What you are looking for in these preliminary searches is the headings in the indexes which deal with your problem. Once you have found these and listed them you should go straight to the Index Medicus and look at that. This is published by the National Library of Medicine U.S.A. and is invaluable for medical and related references. It gives only the titles of papers, classified under subject and also under authors but it does also include books as well as journals. The Index Medicus is available in all Medical School libraries and also in some hospitals. Before you go to the original journals, it may save a good deal of time to look up your titles in some abstracting journal in which you will find a brief summary of the paper. None of the abstracting journals covers all the papers on the subject though ' Excerpta Medica ' is one of the best. A good one is the ' World Abstracts of Medicine ' published by the British Medical Association, ' Psychological Abstracts ' published by the American Psychological Association is very comprehensive for the psychological literature.

If you have found a paper which does give a hint about how to go on further, but is several years old, it is extremely helpful to look at the ' Science Citation Index ', published by the Institute for Scientific Information in Philadelphia, Pennsylvania. You look for this particular paper under the author's name in the Citation Index and there you will find a list of all the works which cite it. These can then be found in full detail, including the title, which is listed under the name of the first author. In this way, having found a lead to further work, you can see if anybody else has done anything about it.

You must work systematically when you are looking up references. Always start with the most recent one that you have and work backwards. When you have found a given reference, always make a proper record of it. Buy yourself a pack of filing cards, the 20 × 15 centimetres size is probably the best, as the smaller ones won't have enough space for what you want to record on them. Copy out the titles of the papers you look up, the authors and the references to them *and make sure you do so accurately*. You should not have to go back to the original papers to make sure that your references are correct. It is a *crime* to give incorrect references! Make careful notes of what you read and put down anything that is relevant to your purpose, put down more rather than less and put down as much detail as you think appropriate. If it turns out that the paper you have read is irrelevant, you should still record its title adding a note that it is of no use to you. This is important. As your work progresses, the number of references you accumulate rapidly increases and you will not remember all of them. Quite easily, you may find yourself going to great trouble to look up a reference and then find you have seen it already. This can happen particularly easily when the only clue to the paper is the name of the author and the reference. It always fills me with fury to see a list of references to a paper which do not include the titles and I resent strongly the spread of this pernicious tendency among medical journals. Full details of references take up space, of course, but a little pruning in the text of the verbiage that passes for English, would provide all that is required.

As you read these papers, you should evaluate them. If they are good, they may give a lead to further work and if they are not then their deficiencies suggest how they can be corrected by new work. Evaluation of published work is difficult but I hope that these lectures will show you how to do it. It is not always difficult; for example, different forms of a disorder, which were previously indistinguishable and can now be differentiated should be considered separately in current research. New methods of diagnosis may mean that older work has become outmoded. Factors now known to be related to onset, course and prognosis may not have been taken into account in the past or you may make a guess that such factors may be relevant and will want to investigate them. The easiest problem of all to tackle is the evaluation of new methods of treatment. In your search of the literature you may wish to find out what are the standard methods for doing so or you may wish to find out how you can improve on them.

MEDLARS

The U.S. National Library of Medicine also issues the Medical Literature Analysis and Retrieval System, known by its acronym as Medlars. This provides a computerized method of finding out references. This may appear to provide a simple solution to your problems, but like all other procedures associated with computers, it may give you more trouble than help, unless you know exactly what to do. The best advice I can give you on using Medlars is to go to a medical librarian and ask her for help. Unless you are very careful, the Medlars system will give you hundreds of titles and since these will all have to be examined you are not really better off than if you had gone directly to the indexes. Medlars can give you references in journals which you are unlikely to know about and if properly used it can cut down enormously the preliminary search and therefore save you much time and effort.

The Unit Hypothesis and Experiment

You will see now that breaking down an investigation into its unit experiments consists not so much of formulating the unit hypothesis as of formulating the unit null hypothesis. It is obvious that when you change your hypothesis you have changed the experiment you are carrying out, but it is equally true that if you alter the null hypothesis then the experiment is changed. The simplest example of this is when you want to investigate the value of a new treatment. If you take a group of subjects who are given the treatment and compare the results with a group of subjects who are not given the treatment, then your null hypothesis is that the treatment does not have any effect. Your investigation will provide you with evidence whether it does. If your experimental treatment is some new therapeutic procedure and you compare its effects with a group of subjects who are given the standard treatment, then your null hypothesis is that there is no difference between treatments and your experiment will tell you if there is. It will not tell you if the new treatment has any affect at all. If the new is better than the standard treatment, then obviously it does have a therapeutic effect; but if it is worse, the experiment cannot tell you whether it has no effect or only a diminished one. You select your control group in order to answer the question you are asking; if you ask another question you select a different control group. The question asked determines the nature of the control group and the null hypothesis and conversely, the nature of the control group determines the null hypothesis and the question you are asking.

Since past experience is not useful and may even be misleading as a measure for evaluating present experience, it is necessary to *make* an appropriate control series. Now when we put in a series of additional cases as controls, what do we get from them? Let us consider the functions of our control series. First of all, it gives us a valid estimation of normal variability or 'error', and this is the basis for the statistical test of significance. In other words, it is the normal variability which gives you the information for determining the probability of the null hypothesis. Secondly, the control series makes the experiment self-contained and therefore it enables us to form our conclusions from the evidence before us.

The valid estimate of error must also be accompanied by an unbiased comparison between contrasted treatments. What does 'unbiased' mean? When I described the simple experiment comparing two treatments on two groups of subjects of five each, I did not say how these subjects were obtained and how they were chosen for the two treatments. If, when you are selecting the subjects for the new treatment, you had selected only the milder cases in order to avoid any risk to them, then clearly the comparison would have been biased. There might be less room for improvement in the milder cases and therefore the new treatment would have appeared to be less effective. Contrariwise, the final state of the milder cases might have been better than the final state of the more serious subjects and therefore the newer treatment would have appeared to be better than the old.

Randomization

The making of a control series is linked with the principle of randomization for there is no point in making a comparison between treatments unless it is an unbiased comparison, and only randomization ensures this. Randomization means that, once a subject is selected as being suitable for inclusion in the investigation, his allocation to a particular treatment, i.e. experimental or control group, is determined solely by chance. Randomization in the experiment is the basis for the application of the theory of probability. When you try to find the probability of the null hypothesis, you do so on the basis of certain theoretical consideration. In order that the theory of probability shall be applicable to the experiment, you must have something within the experiment that corresponds with the theory, and this is the process of randomization. It is this randomization and the theory of error, which constitute the basis for the assumptions underlying the tests of statistical significance. I shall explain this in more detail in a subsequent lecture, and also how randomization is actually carried out.

We know that patients differ considerably in many ways, not only inherently, but in their circumstances. Many of these differences will be factors which will lead, presumably, to the outcome which eventually occurs. The patient will recover, die, improve or not, as the case may be. We can try to identify some of these factors, but we do not know all of them. In the experiment, we deal with the major factors, which produce large effects, by control or selection. The minor and trivial ones which produce only small effects, though they may become big when they accumulate, we try to handle by randomization. We thereby ensure that whichever treatment the patient does eventually receive, he has as good a chance of getting one as the other, and therefore in the long run there will have been as good a chance for the treatments equally to have been given to patients with good and bad prognoses. Then, if the treatments differ in outcome this will show itself as a sort of bias, with better results occurring more frequently for one than the other. For if patients are randomly allotted, then in the long run the outcome will be presumably equal for the two groups, disregarding the treatments. They will tend to be equal, although some patients will do well and some will do ill, so that chance allotments will cause deviations from equality in the groups. Now if one treatment is having a better effect than the other, it will falsify this picture and the corresponding groups will tend to show more and more, that its results are better.

Specification of the Hypothesis

It is not sufficient to take a hypothesis, as at first formulated in indefinite and very general terms, and to restate it in more definite and specific form. It has to be specified and modified until it is in a form which is amenable to experimental attack. This often involves a limitation of the hypothesis.

The investigator has to take account of the circumstances in which he finds himself. He must consider the following three practical problems; subjects, materials and time. First of all he must consider the subjects he has available, what sort of patients. It is a waste of time, when you are in charge of male wards, to try to work on problems which apply to women. It is no good developing theories about genetic psychology or psychoses of children, when you are not working with them. Beginners in research are only too often convinced that the grass is greener in the other fields and I never cease to be astonished at it.

There are other more subtle difficulties. The distribution of age in your patients may be such that certain disorders are uncommon. The location of your hospital may affect the distribution of the social classes of patients who come to it. This may apply in other ways; an obstetric hospital will have many primiparae and multiparae with abnormalities; if you are interested in doing an investigation on normal multiparae you will find that it is the general practitioner who sees them but not the consultant in the obstetric hospital. These are the things on which people fall down most frequently through lack of experience.

Secondly, you have to consider what materials and resources are available. This applies to all sorts of things. I use the term to cover everything, such as machines or other equipment, clinical tests or anything like that. If you are going to do a lot of writing or send a lot of letters, you must have proper clerical facilities. If you have not, do not try that sort of work. If you want to use an electroencephalograph, there must be time available on it to use for the particular purpose and any modifications would require the services of a skilled electronic technician. If you plan to do a biochemical investigation and if you cannot do it yourself, you must find a biochemist who has the time and interest, and so on. It might be very nice to plan some research on drugs which you have heard about; but if they are not available you would be wasting your time.

You must make sure that you have proper facilities for carrying out your research and adequate opportunities to do treatment. There would be no point in planning an investigation on group psychotherapy if the material were not available for it. There might not be a sufficient number of suitable patients, or you may not have sufficient time, or there are no facilities for doing it (I have worked in a hospital where there was not one room available for interviewing patients other than the ward itself). In such cases you cannot do what you want and you must give up the idea.

At the end of your experiment, you will come to the statistical analysis. Here you may be in great difficulty unless you are very careful to think about it beforehand, and ensure that there are sufficient facilities available for computing. It is possible to do statistics the hard way: by hand, with the aid of tables of square and logarithms and your own brains and sweat, not to mention paper and pencils. In such circumstances, you should use only the very simplest of statistical methods, for anything else would just go on and on. If you want anything more elaborate you must plan it carefully on the basis of the facilities available.

Finally, the third thing to be considered is the time available. Most young beginners planning research, and others too, do not have all their free time for it. They are attending training courses, they are doing their routine work, and obviously these must take precedence: they are doctors, after all. They also have a life to live. Some of them have wives who would like to see them sometimes: not too often, just sometimes! Their children would like to see them too. Time is the most expensive and the rarest of all commodities, but it is important from another point of view as well. Obviously, it is no good planning a project of work that would require ten hours a day when you are already doing more or less a full day's work—that is silly. But it is no good planning for follow-up work unless you have time for the follow-up. If one has a job that is to end in one or two years, it is useless to try to do follow-up work which would require five years of observation. For example, I think that in schizophrenia anything less than three to five years of follow-up work is of little value. In cancer, anything less than five years is a waste of time. Even if you plan for a one-year follow-up you must remember that you will not be able to take on any more patients during the last year, and you will have to be certain that you can find enough by that time. So it is no good getting involved in work which will require a longer period than you have available. If you do, you will probably find that your time has been thrown away, for you will not have the opportunity to complete your work later. You may transfer to another job elsewhere with new responsibilities. New interests will develop, it will be difficult to hang on to the old facilities, to find time to do the follow-up work, it will be difficult to get permission to go to your former places, and so on. All these things may arise and the result will be that all the previous efforts are lost.

Available time is sometimes one of the most important factors in deciding which version or form of the hypothesis is going to be dealt with. When one considers, say, the investigation of the effects of a treatment in certain specific conditions, there are different ways of tackling it. You can decide to determine the immediate effects of treatment or the long-term effects, but if you are on a job which is only going to last two or three years, the long-term effects are out of the question and only immediate ones relevant. Remember, a treatment which is not effective by the end of five years, but is effective at the end of one, is not necessarily useless. It may be, for example, that drugs or psychotherapy do not make much difference to the eventual outcome of obsessional states at the end of five years; but either may make a difference in six months or a year's time, and this is not to be despised. For example, cortico-steroids are no better than aspirin for treating rheumatoid arthritis, in the long run, but they may be of great help temporarily. A treatment can be valuable, even if the patient is only partially restored. For a patient to leave a mental hospital for a short while and then return is better than staying there all the time.

It has been pointed out that if you investigate the effects of psychotherapy in the neuroses after a period of years the net results are that two-thirds have recovered or improved greatly and one-third are much the same; and that you find exactly the same results if they have not had any treatment: two-thirds have recovered or improved and one-third are about the same or worse. The effects of intensive psychotherapy and the effects of doing nothing are roughly the same, but this is only in terms of a general outcome in the course of time. The result may be quite different when it comes to a short term investigation or when you consider an immediate return to work. It is not very helpful to a patient to be informed that in five years time he will be back at work and be well again, when he is unemployed at the moment and wants to get back to work right away or within a few months. So one must not despise the short-term investigation however much better a long-term one may be.

Practicability of Design

Here I must mention a point which is a very difficult one, and unhappily not infrequent in medicine. Sometimes, when one is trying to formulate a problem, in order to make it amenable to experimental observation, it may be necessary to reformulate it, to restate one's hypothesis, to make it fit an experimental design that is feasible, rather than the reverse. Ideally, you make some hypothesis and then find a way of tackling it: but sometimes the best way of tackling it may be completely impracticable, so it may be necessary to use another method which is practicable and this may involve reformulating your hypothesis. Obviously this is very unsatisfactory. The experimental method should be subservient to the nature of the problem, but sometimes, life being what it is, it may be necessary to cut the problem down, for example to deal with only one aspect, in order to get some information rather than have none at all. We have chosen between perfection and practicability.

On this matter I can only say what you have heard me say again and again: clinical experiments cannot be designed by experts on experimental design but only by clinicians. You cannot go to a statistician or an expert on experimentation and say ' I want to do some research on this, what is the way to do it?' Even this would be a great improvement on the usual procedure, when the clinician comes along to the statistician and says ' I have gathered a great deal of data, here it is, can you find anything worth while in this pile of stuff? ' or ' How do I analyse this? ' This situation is what makes statisticians burst into tears and go away and hide. It is indeed a bright idea to go to the expert first and ask him how to do a job, but the expert cannot tell you about the clinical aspects of the problem being investigated. Give him a problem, precisely put, then the expert, the statistician, can tell you how it has to be done, but you must get the problem clear in such a way that you *can* have the answer. I would like to add that, in my experience, a detailed discussion with a statistician is a great help even in the earliest stages.

That is the reason why it is important for the clinical investigator to have some idea how experiments are designed, how one sets about a problem, so that he can tackle this necessary first stage. Remember there are no absolute rules for this at all; there cannot be. The rules and principles of experimentation are not at all fixed. They depend on the practical possibilities and, what is more, they depend upon our understanding and the nature of the problems concerned. The principles of experimentation are an aspect of the development of science. What would have been considered an adequate experiment twenty, fifty, a hundred years ago, may not be considered adequate now, and what we think satisfactory now will not be satisfactory in twenty, fifty, or a hundred years' time. Some of the difficulties and problems that have arisen in the course of research have been gradually understood and our ideas on how to tackle them have slowly developed to their present state. But these currently accepted solutions are not infallible, they are not *ex cathedra* statements, they are simply what we understand now at the present stage of science.

Summary

One of the best ways of clarifying a research project is by searching the literature on the subject and in this lecture I have described how this is done. When the problem is defined, it is necessary to break it down into its unit experiments and unit hypotheses. Each one determines the nature of its control group. In order that a control group may serve as the basis for an unbiased comparison, the subjects must be allocated randomly to experimental and control groups.

In planning an experiment, it is necessary to take into account the availability of subjects, materials and time. This is necessary in order to make the experiment practicable.

Experimentation: III

The problem to be investigated having now been selected and, on the basis of various considerations, restricted in scope in a number of ways, it will then be necessary to get down to practical details. Suppose that the hypothesis is that some sort of treatment is likely to be effective, or in the case of the non-therapeutic procedure, is likely to give certain expected results. You have now to plan your experiment and this means that you have to make a number of important decisions. These are practical decisions which must be thought of beforehand and you should write them down clearly and in detail. I have put them under six headings but they are all interdependent. A decision on any one, in a sense, depends on the others.

1. Definition of Treatment

You must first define what you mean by ' treatment '. If you are going to use some form of psychotherapy, you must describe exactly what you mean by it, how much, how often, what sort of psychotherapist and what school of psychotherapy. Is it going to be that of Karen Horney, Alexander and French, Sullivanian, Adlerian, Rogerian or Uncle Tom Cobleigh and all? You may choose freely, but you have to *say what* you have chosen, because whether you get good or bad results, they may or may not be applicable to another kind of psychotherapy. If you are concerned with a drug treatment, you must decide what drug, what dose and what system of administration. I do not have to tell you here that it is one thing to order drugs for a patient, another for the patient to receive them and a third for him actually to swallow them and assimilate them. There's many a slip ' twixt cup and lip '.

There is still much debate about the best method of giving treatments in a clinical trial. Some clinicians believe strongly that the dose should be fixed at some level, to be decided beforehand, and others believe equally strongly that it should vary from patient to patient, or even at different times. In favour of a fixed dose, it can be said that this enables us to standardize the treatment, and since this is a very important factor that will affect our results, we ought to standardize it. There is already sufficient variability among our subjects which we cannot control, without adding another source needlessly. The argument that the dose might be inadequate is dismissed easily, for a trial cannot be conducted without some definite hypothesis based on preliminary investigations and general experience, and this hypothesis includes the dose of treatment.

The real difficulty about a fixed dose is that it might be too much for some patients, since they vary considerably in their sensitivity to the treatment. When this is so, the treatment will tend to produce unpleasant ' side effects ', in which case, if attempts are made to persist with that dose, the patients either will not take it, or will refuse to attend and will therefore be lost from the trial. To keep them in the trial, it will be necessary to reduce the dose, and so the fixed dose has gone.

The method of variable dosage is usually conducted by starting off with a small dose and increasing it until it reaches the maximum that the patient will tolerate. If side-effects appear, the dose is reduced until they disappear. In this way, each patient will receive the maximum tolerable dose of drug, which will thus be given the maximum opportunity of demonstrating its benefits. This is very much like customary clinical practice, and a trial conducted on these lines is therefore very relevant to clinical practice. I am greatly in favour of trials of treatment being conducted in such a way as to make the information obtained of the greatest practical use; I don't see that there is much point in anything else. There is one serious disadvantage of this method and that is that use of an increasing dose tends to produce side-effects. If it is important that the investigator should not know which treatment is being given to a particular patient, the side-effects will reveal which patients are receiving an active drug and which are not (in the case where the controls are receiving a placebo). Where they are receiving another active drug, there may be differences in the side-effects which will reveal which patients are receiving which.

One way of overcoming this is to arrange that the assessments of the condition of the patients should not be made by the physician who is in charge of them and trying to find the appropriate dose for them. This is easier said than done. Even then, patients may complain of side effects when they are being assessed and thus give the game away. There is no doubt that this is a serious difficulty, though as I have just pointed out, it can occur even in the scheme with fixed dosage. I can only say that my experience is that it makes much less difference than one would think. There is no doubt that those who are making the clinical assessments can discover who is taking the active drug, or which one, but they are wrong surprisingly often. Even so, if the assessments are properly (and honestly) done, again it is my experience that any resulting bias is negligible.

No doubt you will have gathered by now that I am in favour of a system of variable dosage; but opinions here are irrelevant. The essential point is that the two schemes of dosage give rise to trials which are concerned with different questions. In the one case the question is ' Is treatment A, given in this particular dose, any better than treatment B (or placebo, as the case may be)?' and in the second case ' Will these patients, when given an optimum dose, do better on the average, with treatment A than with treatment B (or placebo)?'. It seems to me that the point to be decided is which of these questions you are going to ask, and then to plan the trial on that basis. If you look at the problem from that point of view, you will see that sometimes the decision is not in your hands. For example, if the treatment is a new type of operation, then obviously it will be the same for all patients, although presumably the exact details of the operation will vary slightly from patient to patient. If the treatment is a new anaesthetic agent, then clearly it must be given in a dose appropriate to each patient, since there is no other way. If it is an interview under special conditions, it is bound to vary from one subject to another, whatever efforts are made to standardize it.

One could avoid the difficulty between the two alternatives, by dividing the total number of patients into distinct groups which would receive a different level of dose. Within each group the dose would be fixed and at the same time it would be possible to ascertain the effects of such different levels. This does much more than either of the two previous designs, but it has the same disadvantage as the fixed dose scheme, particularly in the higher levels. Undoubtedly, the particular gain from this design is that it settles the question of what is the best dose on the average, but this is a piece of information in which clinicians are rightly not very interested. The disadvantage of this design is that the patients receiving the smaller doses may not show any benefit from the treatment, so they are effectively lost from the trial, which is wasteful. I have already mentioned that those receiving the higher doses may drop out and thus lead to waste at the other end.

Another question that is often asked, is ' Should patients receive any supplementary treatments during the trial?' I have little doubt that you know the answer I give to this inquiry: it depends on the question you are asking. Supplementary treatments can be included as indicated for each patient, or they may be given systematically.

2. Population (what sort of patients)

I have already pointed out that a report describing an investigation is an historical document describing a past event. Its significance lies in the future. If the investigation showed that a certain treatment was effective, the practicing clinician will want to know on what sort of patients it was effective in order that he can make use of this treatment on other patients. It is assumed that the group on which the investigation was carried out is not unique, that there are other patients with similar characteristics. The experimental group can therefore be regarded as a sample from a ' population '. The information we have obtained from this group is going to be applied to other groups or samples from this population. This group is therefore regarded as being representative of the population; and as I shall show later, this is fundamental in the statistical analysis. In treating this group as representative we are faced with a problem which is not quite as simple as it looks. We do our investigation on patients in a particular hospital, and if it comes to that, we do not do it on patients in the hospital, we do it on those in a particular ward or group of wards, and then we believe, or hope, that what has happened to those patients can be assumed to be relevant to other patients in the hospital, to other patients in the city, to others in the country and to others elsewhere, all over the world. You see that at each phase of the extension of the notion of what the population is, we are on more and more dangerous ground. We must beware of extending our inferences to the bigger group until we are quite certain where we stand. If we are not quite certain we must state this. It is therefore necessary to describe the relevant characteristics of the group in such a way that the population from which it is derived is clearly recognizable.

Some characteristics are standard; for example, you always describe the age and sex. In America and some other countries it is customary to mention the proportion of coloureds and whites. In some countries you may find that religion is very important. Social class is generally considered a relevant factor in describing the patients and it may be so. It may be fairly important for out-patients, it is very important for new admissions but I do not think it matters very much for patients who have been in hospital for ten or twenty years. By this time their social class is quite simply defined as ' chronic hospital patient ', regardless of the other categories. These characteristics must be defined. Remember, what is relevant for one group, may be irrelevant for another.

At this stage it is important to consider carefully the suitability of the type of the subjects which have been chosen for your particular inquiry. It is obvious that the type should be appropriate, but what this may mean in any particular instance is not always easy to say. Sometimes, it is not so much the patients as the disorder or treatment that has to be selected carefully. I am reminded of the surgeon who investigated a drug which was alleged to diminish the tendency to develop oedema after injury. Very ingeniously, he and his colleague tested the drug by giving it to patients who had had surgical operations that were known to induce oedema easily, such as operations near the eye. Obviously, it would be very difficult to test the value of the drug if the patients were unlikely to show oedema even without it. I may add that the investigation was carefully conducted, with proper controls and so on.

In the same way, if you wanted to test the effect of an analgesic you would have to make sure that you were dealing with a type of painful condition which was unlikely to disappear or rather, in which it was reasonable to expect the pain to continue for the period of observation. Otherwise, you would be faced with the problem that some of the cases which showed diminished pain, or even disappearance of the pain, did so because of the natural process of recovery. Of course, if you have a control series, and you have properly allotted your patients to either of the groups (by ' randomization ') the value of the analgesic will show itself in the differences between the two groups; but because of the natural remission, you will need to have many more cases in the series. Similarly, if you were testing a treatment to prevent premenstrual tension, you would choose patients whose history showed that they could be expected to have the symptoms without fail, if untreated.

WIDE OR NARROW GROUPS

This immediately presents you with the problem that the group you are investigating may be a very limited one, and one which is not at all representative of the general run of patients. In coping with this, you are always faced with a choice between two opposite difficulties. If you limit your investigation to a narrowly defined group of cases, then, since the group consists of individuals very much alike in the limiting (and presumably important) characteristics, the homogeneity of your group gives rise to great consistency or response. The natural variation between individuals is diminished in your groups and this means that you can obtain your result with a relatively small number of cases. Obviously this makes the investigation shorter and involves less work, though you may find yourself in difficulties in trying to find enough patients in your limited category. Unfortunately, the limitation of the type of case also limits the range of your conclusions, since your conclusions can apply only to that type of patient. Thus, if your patients were men, over 40 years, and showing a loss of weight of over four kilos, then your conclusions will not help you in dealing with a young woman who has not lost weight, or even a young man who has.

The opposite difficulty arises when you make few limitations in the type of patient. Although it is easier to find suitable patients, for then all is grist to your mill, the great variability among them means that you will have to have many more patients in your groups. It is true that your results will have more general applicability, but this is a very superficial way of looking at things. The results of your investigation will merely tell you that you will tend to get better results with treatment A than treatment B. With both treatments you will have successes and failures, but when you are dealing with individual patients, you want to know which ones will be successes and which will be failures. It is true that you can look at the failures and successes in your investigation, and decide that they differ in certain ways. This is sometimes done, and these observations are then treated as if they were conclusions derived from the data. This is quite mistaken. An experiment can give answers to the questions it was designed to test, and to those only. It can give you information on your specific hypotheses and to no others. Any additional observations you make during the course of the experiment can be used to formulate new hypotheses, but these must be tested in an experiment designed for that purpose. This is a very common error, even in investigations which have been very well designed. This is the point I made in an earlier lecture: that the conclusions do not follow from the data.

Another aspect of this difficulty is that among your subjects are different types of person, or of disorder, of which only one type, or a limited number, respond to the treatment, and the others do not. If the 'responsive' types are relatively few in number, then they may be swamped by the large number of cases that do not respond to the treatment, and so you may obtain a null result. For example, if you were to test the value of liver in the treatment of anaemia, you could easily obtain a null result, even if you tried it on a hundred or more cases, for iron deficiency anaemia, which is not responsive to liver, is very common, and Addisonian anaemia, which is responsive, is comparatively rare. Of course, such an experiment would never be done, because we have been able to distinguish between these radically different diseases very easily, and for long before we knew of the value of liver. But in many other disorders the only way in which we can distinguish between the different varieties is that some patients do respond to treatment and others do not. If we do not know how to distinguish these types, we do not know how to estimate the proportions of these types in any given series of patients, so that we cannot be sure that one series is comparable with another. This is simply another way of explaining why we have to have a control series, and why an experiment has to be self-contained. If we take our series of cases, and ' randomly ' allot them to two or more treatments, then we can be sure that any differences in the proportion of responsive to unresponsive case will follow the laws of chance, so that our test of significance will be meaningful.

REACTION TO PLACEBO

The effects of a treatment tend to be obscured not only by the ' spontaneous ' recoveries, but also by the type of patient who responds to any form of ' treatment ', i.e those who react to a placebo. Obviously, we can overcome this difficulty by taking enough cases in our investigation, but there is no doubt that the reactions to placebo tend to obscure the effectiveness of the active treatment. In the more general cases, we can tackle this problem and improve the effectiveness of our investigation, by eliminating those cases who will recover anyway, and including those who will not.

There are two ways in which we can endeavour to eliminate the ' placebo reactor '. We can start by giving all patients a placebo, and eliminating from the trial of treatments those who respond to it, or we can use a ' cross-over ' design, i.e. one in which all patients receive the active treatment and the placebo, one or the other first, and then eliminate those who have responded both to the active treatment and to the placebo. The difficulty with the first method is that the investigator knows that all the patients are receiving a placebo, and it would appear that one of the ingredients for the response to placebo is a sufficient enthusiasm for the treatment on the part of the physician. This does not always apply, and too much should not be made of it, but the problem does exist. Underlying both methods is the assumption that reaction to placebo is a constant characteristic of the patient, and this is not necessarily true. There is much confusion on this subject, and assertions that the patient who reacts to a placebo has a distinct type of personality are countered by statements that such reactions depend upon the therapist, the therapeutic situation and all sorts of environmental circumstances. Sometimes these two assertions will be made consecutively by the one individual! A fair amount of research has been done on this problem, but it is still far from being settled. The determinants of the behaviour of a given human being in a particular situation are among the most complex phenomena we are likely to meet, and it is rather naïve to think that behaviour can be made simple by labelling it ' placebo reactions '.

My remarks so far have implied that an active treatment is being compared with a placebo or dummy treatment given to the ' control ' group, but with suitable modifications it applies equally to the cases where two actvie treatments are being compared. If the less active one gives good results, it will be all the more difficult to demonstrate that the more active treatment is better, and the investigator will have to use large groups of patients. We can alter the investigation by picking that type of patient which is not likely to react well to the standard treatment, and this will certainly cut down the number of patients required to evaluate the treatment, but I am sure that you will recognize immediately that you have changed the hypothesis by changing the experiment. Instead of asking whether the new treatment is better than the old, you are now asking if the new treatment is effective in those patients for whom the old treatment is not. This is quite a different question, for it is always possible that the new treatment may be effective only where the old one was, but more so. I hope that I am not giving the impression that I am concerned with minor subtleties, or mere ' logic chopping '. These are very practical problems. For example, to try out a new treatment for diabetes mellitus on insulin-resistant diabetics is a very different matter from trying it out on the general run of diabetics.

3. Selection of a Criterion

Surprising as it may seem, this is sometimes forgotten, or rather, dealt with very haphazardly. If you are going to investigate the value of a treatment how do you decide if it is any good or not? What is your decision based upon? I am not going to lay down the law about good and bad criteria. This has to be decided in each particular investigation, but it must be decided beforehand and not halfway through or at the end. I need not dwell on the need for the criterion to be sensitive to the changes expected. Furthermore, it must be clearly defined. You can, if you wish, say that a patient will be classified as 'recovered' when you say he has recovered, and 'not recovered' when you say he has not. You can do it that way if you like, but it is always possible to say on what grounds you make these decisions, and it is very useful if you can give grounds that are clearly recognized by everybody. When describing your work give examples which show how the grounds have been used in making these decisions, so that everybody can recognize them and see that you have made them properly. If you do no more than say 'what I say three times is true', i.e. if I say the patient has recovered he has recovered, and vice versa, then your reader has to decide whether he is interested in your opinion or not. If he is, he goes on reading, but if he is not, he turns over the page and that's that.

Before a criterion can be defined, it must first be selected, and there are many difficulties here. When you compare two treatments, it is possible that a null result may be obtained because the method of measuring the criterion is incapable of showing differences. Even if it does show them, these may be regarded by others as trivial or irrelevant. You have measured the differences between the treatments in one way, but this is not the way that matters. That may be very obvious when you know what matters, but you don't always know, or others may disagree with you. For example, if you want to compare two treatments for angina pectoris, do you test them by their effects on the ECG or by the response of the patients to exercise? Do you test treatments for hypertension by their effects on the blood pressure, or on the patient's symptoms, or by the long-term development of complications? When we discuss the effects of a treatment for neurosis, do we mean the change in symptoms, the change in social behaviour, or the change in psycho-dynamics (the brand specified)? We are always faced with the possibility of this sort of criticism, and we must be prepared to justify our choice of criterion.

When we design an experiment, we are faced with the problem that the specification of the hypothesis we are testing, and its accompanying null hypothesis is not at all obvious. To state it requires a knowledge of the background subject matter of the experiment, even a good deal of knowledge. For example, when dealing with the treatment of asthma we have to know that there are two kinds of asthma; the first type tends to appear at a very early age in childhood, goes on into adult life into the twenties and then usually fades away. This type is extremely sensitive to emotional changes in the patients. There is a second type of asthma which appears in late life, the forties and fifties. It is severe, is very recalcitrant to treatment, responds very little to emotional changes in the patient, and can be fatal. Anybody who investigates the treatment for asthma must differentiate clearly between these two kinds and must define quite clearly the nature of his question and the null hypothesis. If, for example, he is dealing with the first type he is not going to get very much further if he delays evaluation of the treatment until the patients are, say, twenty-five to thirty, and his criterion is recovery. Most of such patients will have recovered anyway. Contrariwise, if he is going to determine the effect of, shall we say, psychotherapy, he is not going to get very far if he uses the second type which is unresponsive to it. If he mixes the two types in one group, his results, whatever he does, will depend chiefly on the proportions of the two types.

If you want to investigate the treatment for duodenal ulcer, it is important to recognize that duodenal ulcer is a recurrent disorder. Every patient who gets an attack can be assured with fair certainty that he will recover from it. There is no difficulty here. Unfortunately you can also tell him, with regretful assurance, that he is likely to get another attack in due course. Therefore when we set up an experiment for the treatment of duodenal ulcer it is inadequate to base our hypothesis, about the effectiveness of the treatment, on the criterion of recovery from the attack; and to make the null hypothesis the statement that the patients will not recover from the attack, because they do. The null hypothesis is not simple in such cases, it needs careful thinking to decide what we are out to achieve and what will be a blank result. It must be recognized that a statistician cannot advise on these points. He can give advice on statistics, but not on the subject-matter and the difficulty of the material concerned. It is therefore very important for the experimenter himself to know these problems, and to understand something about the design of experiments and their statistical analysis.

4. Experimental Control

The factors to be controlled in the experiment have to be identified. Here we come back to the point that I have made repeatedly. *You* have to decide what factors within your population are likely to make an important difference to the results of treatment. For example if you are working on a re-educative program, say, on chronic patients, you must consider carefully whether you think that this program will work with greater difficulty on patients who have been in hospital a long time as compared with those who have been recently admitted, or vice versa. If you decide that the length of stay in hospital would be likely, on the basis of your knowledge, experience and theories, to play an important part in the results, then you must make up your mind what you are going to do about it. You can decide to standardize length of stay by taking your patients from a narrow-range group; in this way you eliminate the effects of length of stay. If all your subjects have been in hospital for ten years then it will not be possible to tell whether lesser or greater stay in hospital makes any difference to the results. You have wiped it out of the experiment by standardizing. At the same time you have ensured that it is not going to interfere with your results, because one group has a shorter and the other a longer stay. There are other ways of dealing with this problem as I shall explain in due course but the point is that you must consider it beforehand. 'Is this important, am I going to bother with it and if so, what am I going to do about it?

5. Final Restatement of the Problem

Having defined your treatments, your population, your criterion and your factors, you now restate the problem, this time in specific terms. You do not ask 'Does this treatment work?', you now ask if the treatment, given in such-and-such a way, by such persons, under such conditions, to patients of the following type and nature, produces any improvement, as observed, measured or recorded by the following criteria, taking into account such factors as age, sex and so on. This final restatement of the problem should always be made. Sit down and write it out quite explicitly. In some institutions it is customary to demand a 'research protocol', which is an excellent training for this purpose. It forces the individual to put down in black and white, in coherent, grammatical sentences, precisely what he is after, instead of thinking vaguely that he is going to do something or other, and hope for the best.

When you are working out your experiment and the questions you are trying to investigate, it is very important to consider all likely alternative results and their interpretation. Before you start, you should consider every possible result that you can get or could conceivably get and what inferences you would draw from them. You must use your imagination here and you must use it as far as possible to anticipate the confusion and difficulties that will assail your investigation if they are not foreseen. If you do not think of these difficulties and do something about them, they will appear in the course of the experiment and because you have not dealt with them they may invalidate your conclusions. It is certain that other people who read your work will find them. It is therefore necessary, at the beginning of an experiment, to examine it very carefully to test it, to try to tear it to pieces.

All of these difficulties must be thought of beforehand, and this is very tricky. It needs experience, a detailed knowledge of the clinical material, of the material with which you are working and of the field with which you are concerned. This again is something that only the experimenter can do, and nobody else can. Whatever field you are working in, medicine, surgery, nursing, psychiatry or social work, only those actually involved can understand the problems and difficulties that will arise. You can anticipate these difficulties, or you can wait until the end of the experiment and have others point them out to you; and remember, your critics will know them very well.

6. Experimental Design

When we have this final statement of the problem, under specific conditions, we come to the last item, the selection of a specific experimental design. I make this the last of the decisions, for I have to put them in some order (since I cannot list all six types simultaneously), but they are closely intertwined. When I dealt with the control of factors, I was already talking of the experimental design; so too with the selection of criteria. When you consider these points, you deal with them more or less simultaneously, each modifying the other until you get to the final point: consideration of a specific experimental design.

It is here that the expert, the statistician, can give you advice.

That is the point I want to bring out. Of the six decisions you have to make before you can start an experiment the statistician can give you advice on only one: selection of the experimental designs; but any one of the other five subjects is just as important. He cannot tell you what you mean by treatment and the dose and method of administration; the definition of the population is not his concern. You can test your treatment on senile dements or on adolescent youths; it is for you to decide what you are going to do; he cannot advise. The statistician cannot devise a criterion, for only you, only the clinician, knows what is meant by improvement or recovery. If you do not, nobody else does. The statistician might be able to give you some advice on the identification of the factors to be controlled, but not often.

The selection of a specific experimental design is only one of your many problems, but I do not want to lean over backwards and suggest it is unimportant. On the contrary, for one of the things we always have to bear in mind is that we are not doing experiments out of idle curiosity, merely as a way of passing the time. We are hoping to make a contribution to knowledge, and also—it may sound priggish, but it is true—we are hoping that our efforts will contribute to the relief of human suffering. To do this we want to get as clear results as possible and as speedily as possible; for on the one hand, we do not want to withhold a good treatment from patients longer than is necessary, and, on the other hand, and this is equally important, we do not want to disseminate the use of an unnecessary, dangerous, or useless treatment and expose people to it. We need an answer to our investigation as quickly as possible, using the minimum number of patients for the minimum amount of time. This is where the statisticians have the answers. The question of the efficiency of experiments, getting the maximum amount of information from the minimum amount of material, is just what they have been working on, and they know how to squeeze the last drop of juice from your orange. But whether it is a ripe orange or a rotten one, only you can decide.

All of the things I have been talking about take time, a considerable amount of time, and they should never be rushed. I have boasted that in one investigation I did, it took me over nine months to get started on my first patients (excluding the preliminaries). This is lengthy but it is not excessive. You cannot plan an investigation in a few weeks or even a month or two. Take plenty of time to go into these points and settle them. Remember this, and it is the last thing I have to say now: it is important to get the maximum criticism at the start of an experiment. Take your time, go and get advice, ask people to pull it to pieces. You cannot have enough criticism at the beginning of the experiment; it is at the end, when you have completed your work and someone points out that it is fallacious or has flaws, that criticism really hurts.

Summary

The planning of an experiment requires decisions and detailed specification of six interdependent problems. Definition of treatment includes also supplementary treatments. Description of population includes methods of sampling and the inclusion of wide or narrow gaps. Special consideration has also to be given to coping with placebo-reaction. The selection of a suitable criterion of change can be difficult and requires clinical judgement. Factors affecting results may have to be excluded or controlled. All these may require re-formulation of the original hypothesis. Finally, a suitable design for the experiment has to be chosen.

REFERENCE

CALMAN, J. & BARR, A. (1960). The prevention of post-operative oedema. *British Medical Journal,* **ii,** 261-263.

The Design of Experiments

Let me remind you about the stages of experimentation. The second is to form a clear and defined hypothesis. The third is to design an experiment which will answer the question raised in the hypothesis, and this will be the subject of this lecture. The experiment will provide a set of data which will have to be submitted to statistical analysis. It is this analysis which enables you to draw conclusions about the original hypothesis. In the language of statistics, the experiment should be so designed that there are two hypotheses: your original one, the positive hypothesis, and its alternative, the null hypothesis.

The subject of the design of experiments has become extraordinarily complex, and a glance at a standard text-book on the subject can be very frightening to the enquiring clinician. I confess that sometimes I begin to think that the subject has become a branch of pure mathematics: I find it very difficult to imagine what sort of experiment could require a 10×10 Graeco-Latin-square design. The mathematical statistician could reply to this that my lack of imagination was my misfortune, but not his problem!

The clinical investigator need know only the more elementary designs at present, and it is likely to be a long time before he will need more. I venture the safe prediction that the greatest developments in clinical medicine will, for a long time, depend on advances in basic sciences of medicine, rather than on the development of techniques in clinical research. I am not thereby decrying clinical research, for the discoveries of basic science will eventually have to be applied and tested in clinical practice. 'The proof of the pudding is in the eating'.

THE MYTH OF 'LARGE NUMBERS'

When the beginner has realized that he will have to do a statistical analysis on his data, he is apt to think that this means that he will have to investigate a large number of cases—a frightening prospect. This is a mistaken notion. Some investigations may need large numbers of cases, but the majority of clinical investigations do not. In the first place, the statistical test of significance takes into account the number of cases you have, and will indicate what conclusion you can draw from that number; but this is only a minor point. The important thing to remember is that a few cases carefully investigated will give more useful information than a large number badly or carelessly observed. If you are interviewing patients, then a few careful, detailed, leisurely interviews are better than many short sessions consisting of little more than a few brief questions hurled at the patient and noted down in a hurry. A relatively small number of EEG records, done carefully and of sufficient length, will generally be better than numerous short records, which may easily lack precisely what you are looking for. Even if you are doing some chemical test, it may be better to use an elaborate time-consuming procedure a few times, rather than a simple test many times, if the latter is inaccurate. Of course, great accuracy or detail may be unnecessary, it all depends what you are trying to do, but it is a general rule that it is the quality of your observations that should be good, rather than that the quantity should be great.

Furthermore, if an experiment is badly done so that it is not meaningful, if it is done in such a way that various unknown factors are introducing a bias into the experiment, then it doesn't matter whether you do it on ten patients, a hundred or a thousand. It is still biased and the experiment is still bad. The only difference is that it may be said that a hundred cases are five times more deluding and misleading than twenty. There is no safety in numbers.

At this point many of you are beginning to think that ' relatively small ' or ' relatively large ' numbers are rather vague statements. How does one decide how many patients should be investigated? As I shall deal with this in detail in due course, I shall content myself with the brief statement that it all depends on what sort of result you expect to obtain. If the difference between your two groups, say treated and untreated, is likely to be large, then you will need only a few cases to demonstrate that difference, and vice versa. How can you know beforehand how big a difference you can expect? The ' trial run ', which is the first stage of your investigation, will tell you this.

THE MYTH OF ' ONE VARIABLE '

What is an experiment? Our idea of the essential features of an ' experiment ' is comparatively modern and comes from Galileo.

He taught that in order to investigate a particular system, the experimenter has to standardize the experimental situation, i.e. he has to hold constant all the factors that may affect the behaviour of the system, and then alter one of them, the significant one which he is investigating, and thereby determine its effect by seeing how the system alters in response to the change. When the experimenter alters one factor, or, in modern terminology, changes one ' input ' into the system, then this becomes the ' cause ' of this change in the system, which is the ' effect '. One can still read statements that this is the essence of the experimental method: hold all the factors constant and then alter one at a time. This may have been a reasonable description of experimental method in the past, but it is certainly mistaken nowadays. In the first place, it is not always easy to say which is the significant factor, and this is particularly true of biological phenomena. In the second place, we cannot be certain that the effects of the one factor are independent of the others; or, at best, related to them in some simple way. The effect of one factor may depend on the conditions, i.e. the other factors. For example, we know now that the effect of a dose of vaccine on immunity will depend not only on whether a previous dose has been given, but when it was given. Thus the experimenter who restricts himself to altering only one factor at a time may be losing very important information.

It was that great genius Ronald Fisher who broke the bounds of the Galilean system of experimentation and showed how it was possible to alter more than one factor at a time and yet to disentangle from the results the effect of each individual factor. Not only that, but he was able to show how the interaction between factors, the way they influence each other, could be found. I am sure that in the history of experimental science, the name of Fisher will rank with that of Galileo, and I am always surprised how little this is recognized even by those who ought to understand the significance of Fisher's contribution. I shall explain Fisher's ideas in due course but let us first start with an example.

Simple Design

Let us suppose that a surgeon has been offered a new drug, on which there is evidence that it will destroy cancer cells. He decides to try it on cases of cancer of the breast. Of course, he will operate on all his patients, but he would like to find out if the drug is better than radiotherapy as a supplement to the operation. He decides to set about it as follows: he takes a series of cases, as they come, and randomly allots them by spinning a coin or some equivalent method, to either of the two treatments, radiotherapy (treatment R) or drug (treatment D), say 60 each. It is desirable to have equal numbers in each group so the cases are allotted randomly until 60 cases have had one treatment, and then all the rest have the other, up to 60. The reason for equality of numbers in the groups is that this gives the maximum amount of information for a given total number of subjects. In this way, he will compare the effectiveness of the two supplementary treatments, with 60 cases in each group, the total coming to 120. On further consideration, he decides that since both of these treatments entail some risk to the patients, which may or may not outweigh its advantages, he will test whether the supplementary treatments have any overall advantage over the operation alone, so he decides to allot his patients to three groups, 40 in each, one of which will not receive a supplementary treatment after operation. (How does one allot patients to three groups by spinning a coin? It can be done, but it is easier to carry out the allocation by throwing dice. The six faces of a die are allocated to the three treatments and the patient allocated according to the face which comes up. An easier way, when one knows how, is to use a table of random numbers.) Table 7.1.

TABLE 7.1

Treatment O	40
Treatment R	40
Treatment D	40
Total number of cases	120

The set-up is as in Table 7.1, calling the no-supplement group as treatment O. The difference between the results of treatment R and treatment O gives him the effect of treatment R, on 40 cases. In the same way he can determine the effect of treatment D, also on 40 cases. Finally, he can compare treatments R and D on 40 cases. He has lost something, because of the decrease in the size of his groups from 60 to 40, but he has gained because he can now obtain the answers to three questions instead of to one.

This simple experiment, comparing the effect of one supplementary treatment against a 'control' series not receiving it, enables him to answer one question: the value of that supplement. Repeating the experiment with the other supplement enables him to answer a second question: the value of the other. Combining the two experiments enables him to answer a third question: the relative merits of the two supplements. Why can the two separate experiments not answer the third question? That was dealt with in the earlier lectures on the 'self-contained' experiment. Combining the two experiments has also led to economy in the number of 'control' cases. The original design required 120 patients to answer one question. Even if the number of cases in the three groups is increased to 60 each, there is still a gain in efficiency, because three questions can now be answered with the 180 cases.

Factorial Design

So far, the design of the experiment follows the principle of altering only one factor at a time: either a patient has one supplement or the other. This is an unnecessary restriction, however, and the experiment could be done in the following way (Table 7.2):

TABLE 7.2

Treatment O	30
Treatment R	30
Treatment D	30
Treatment R + D	30
Total number of cases	120

To determine the effect of treatment R, the surgeon can not only compare the results of treatment R against treatment O, 30 cases, but also the effect of treatment R + D against treatment D, 30 cases, giving a total of 60 cases for the comparison. In the same way, he can determine the effects of treatment D by comparing it with treatment O and comparing treatment R + D with treatment R, again 60 cases. Furthermore, he can now determine whether the two treatments combined are better than either of them alone, for 30 of his cases have had the two together. Notice that not only is the number of cases required the same as before, but for determining the effects of treatments R and D he has gone back to the original size of the groups, a rise from 40 to 60.

The design of this experiment is easier to follow if we regard the supplement as being in two doses or intensities, absent or present.

We can then illustrate it in the form of a square diagram, Fig. 7.1 :

	O	R	Total
O	(Treatment 0) ('controls') 30	Treatment R 30	60
D	Treatment D 30	Treatment R + D 30	60
Total	60	60	120

Figure 7.1. Two-way factorial design.

The simple combination of two experiments increased the number of questions that could be answered from one to three; but by combining the experiments in a factorial design, the answer to a fourth question can be obtained: the value of the interaction between the supplementary treatments. Furthermore, this is done, not by decreasing but by increasing the numbers in the groups compared. We see that the factorial design is the most efficient here.

It is important to be clear about what lies behind this design. When we examine the difference between group R and O we have as our background the null hypothesis that the difference between the two is no greater than would be found by chance if we took groups of individuals by random sampling. If the null hypothesis has a probability so low that we reject it then we are justified in assuming that the difference between these two groups is due to treatment R. The same applies when we compare group (R + D) with group D (and this is true regardless of whether treatment D is found to have a real effect, i.e. we rejected the null hypothesis that the differences between those groups given D and those not, is due to chance). The argument applies equally when we make comparisons in the columns, i.e. when we compare group D against group O and group (R + D) against group R. If you think it over, you will see that it is implied that whatever may be the causes of the difference between individuals in any one group, the effect of treatment R on its group is merely to increase the criterion score, i.e. the effect of R is added on to the normal variation between individuals. The same applies to treatment D and also for both treatments occurring together. This assumption, that the effects of treatments are additive, is basic to the notion of the factorial design and its statistical analysis. Of course, it may not be true, but then the evidence of its falsity will be found in the data and be demonstrated by the statistical analysis.

When we examine the data to determine the effect of treatment R, then, in the top row, group O serves as the base line or control series for group R. In the bottom row group D also serves as such a base line, despite the fact that treatment D may have had some effect. The design of the experiment has this result therefore, that by subtraction we can eliminate the difference between group D and group O so that both can serve as a control series. This notion, that we can subtract the effects of one factor in order to examine the effects of another is fundamental to this design and to its statistical analysis.

THREE FACTORS IN TWO STAGES

The number of factors to be varied in the experiment can be increased indefinitely beyond two. For the case of three factors, the design can best be shown by changing the square to a cube, Fig. 7.2:

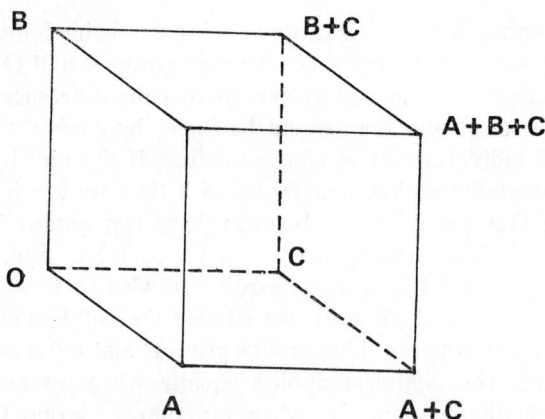

Figure 7.2. Three-way factorial design in two levels each.

Four factors can be represented by two cubes, each one of which represents the fourth factor at one of its levels. Very elaborate layouts are required to represent more factors.

The factorial design may be used not only for experimental

factors which are under the control of the experimenter, but also for observational data which classify the patients into categories. Thus, in the diagram of the cube above, A can represent age (O subjects are young and A are old), B can be sex (O are Women and B are men) and C can represent severity of illness (O are mild and C are severe). The same treatment is given to all the patients, or the same observation made on them, and the relation between the results of treatment and the 'factors' and their interactions obtained.

A very neat example of this particular design has been used for evaluating the effects of stilboestrol, phenobarbitone and 'gastric diet' in the treatment of chronic duodenal ulcer. The three factors were the two different drugs and the diet. Each had two ordinary levels: placebo against adequate dose for the drugs, and ordinary diet against a gastric one. The design is illustrated in Figure 7.3.

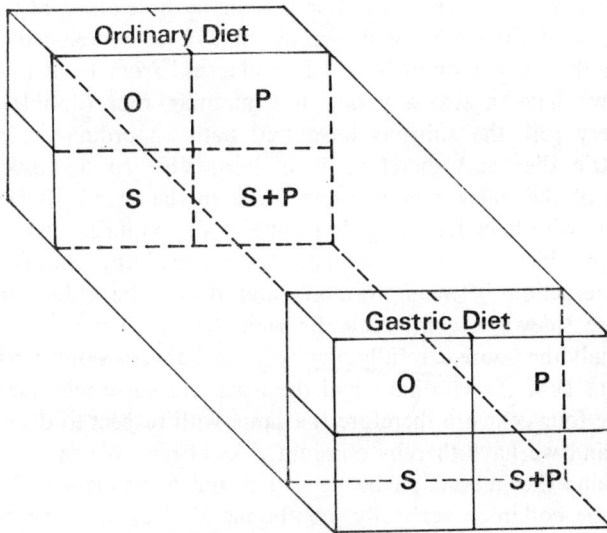

Figure 7.3. Trial of gastric diet, phenobarbitone and stilboestrol for treatment of duodenal ulcer.

The cube which illustrates this three-way factorial design has been separated into two slabs, the rear slab consists of those subjects on an ordinary diet and the front slab of those on a gastric diet. The corresponding cells in each slab have the same combination of drugs. To compare the effect of special diet versus ordinary diet we compare the results of the cases in the front slab with those in the rear slab. To determine the effects of phenobarbitone we compare the right-hand columns against the left-hand columns and to compare the effect of stilboestrol we compare the lower halves of both slabs with the upper halves. In this way we evaluate the 'main effects'.

When a subject receives two or more treatments, the effect of each treatment may appear regardless (independent) of the effects of the others. In that case, the effects of the treatments will be additive. Alternatively, the two treatments may inhibit or potentiate each other's effects so that the net result of both is not the same as the sum of the two. This is what is meant by 'interaction'. I have already pointed out how a two-way design provides the information for determining the interactions between two factors. How is this done for a three-way design? It is done by converting the three-way to a two-way design and this is done in three different ways. If you look at Figure 7.3 you can see that if we combine the front slab with the rear one (the cube 'collapses' from front to back), then we have a two-way design containing four (double) cells. In every cell, the subjects have had both an ordinary diet and a gastric diet and therefore it is impossible to determine the effects of the differences between diets. In the four cells we have subjects who have had drug, hormone, both combined and neither. This provides us with the data for determining the effect of the interaction between hormone and drug. The cube can also collapse sideways, combining the right half with the left half. If you study the figure carefully, you will see that each double cell now contains subjects who have had the drug and some who have not. All the four cells are therefore the same with respect to drug treatment and we have thereby eliminated its effects. We can therefore determine the interaction between diet and hormone. Similarly, if the cube collapses vertically, combining the top and the bottom half, we can determine the interaction between drug and diet. In the statistical analysis of the data, we determine the three main effects, the three two-way interactions and then subtract these from the overall effects thus leaving us with the three-way interaction between drug, diet and hormone. This will be easier to follow when we come to work out an actual example but it is important to try and understand the logic behind the statistical technique.

A similar design but more complicated because one of the factors has three ' levels ' is exemplified by an investigation in which I was involved. The effects of two drugs, prochlorperazine (PCP) and trifluoperazine (TFP) were compared against each other and against no drug (P). At the same time, intensive nursing and social rehabilitation (for which the old term ' moral treatment ' was revived) was compared with routine care (RC). The patients were classified into three groups according to their deterioration, moderate, marked and severe. This was done on male and female patients separately. The drugs, including the blank, form one factor; the ' moral treatment ' (MT) and routine care are the second factor; severity of deterioration is the third, and sex is the fourth. Once the experiment had been set up, the data on the initial state of the patients was examined, and this showed that the condition of the female patients was not comparable with that of the males. The four-way design had therefore, to be separated into two separate three-way experiments. The three grades of patients had to be put into three separate wards (which introduced some complications), and as the smallest ward could hold only 21 patients, the total number of patients was 63 each of the two sexes. The structure of the experiment is illustrated in Figure 7.4.

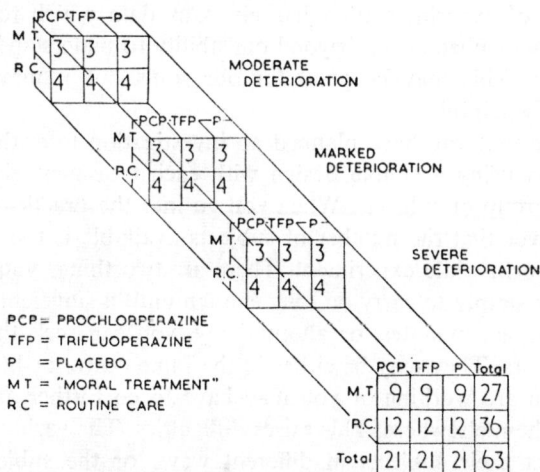

Figure 7.4. Three-way factorial design : 2 × 3 × 3 levels.

The factorial design can be further elaborated by increasing the number of stages or levels of each factor. Thus a treatment could be given in small, medium or large dose, age could be divided into a series of ranges, and so on. The 'levels' of each factor need not necessarily be in quantitative form. Thus, one of the factors could be the four main blood-groups.

There is no theoretical limit to the complexity of a factorial design, but there are many practical limitations. A very elaborate design requires a very large number of cases, since one must have at least two cases in each 'cell' of the design, and two is a very small number. A large number of cases entails much work for a long time before the experiment is completed and before any results are available. When the factor is made up of observational categories, one may be held up for months looking for, say, two or more women between the ages of 50 to 59 years, of blood group AB and suffering from the disease in a mild form. At the end, it may turn out that the variation in some of the factors was unnecessary, since they made no difference, and all that time and work has been lost. Of course, the subjects have not been lost; the experiment has merely included more subjects than were absolutely necessary. In practice, it is better to start off with some simple design and use its results to indicate the direction for further investigations.

One of the troubles with complex designs is that when complex interactions are found, it is very difficult to interpret them. The technique of experimentation has given us data which reveal the complexity of phenomena beyond our ability to understand or deal with them. This may be good for our souls but it may not be particularly helpful.

Suppose that you have planned an investigation to evaluate two treatments, using a simple design with each treatment given to a separate group of subjects. When you go into the practical details, you discover that the number of subjects available is too small to make a worth-while experiment. There are two things you can do, the first is simply to carry on long enough until a sufficient number of subjects accumulates, or alternatively, you can seek the aid of collaborators. They may be either in the same centre or hospital in which you are working or you may have to go further afield and look for them elsewhere. This raises difficulties. The various centres may select their subjects in different ways, or the subjects may differ in social or environmental circumstances. Furthermore, the methods of assessment may differ; their laboratories may use different techniques or have different standards. At each centre the same simple design will be used but at every one the number of subjects will be insufficient. You will therefore have to combine the data from all the centres, but if there are differences between the centres, then there will be an increase in the variability in the groups and this will increase the probability of the null hypothesis. You may therefore find that you have lost as much as you have gained.

The way to deal with this is to consider ' centres ' as a factor and thereby convert your simple two-group experiment into a two-way factorial design. The statistical analysis will enable you to eliminate the effects of the centres, and enable you to examine the effects of treatment as if all subjects had come from one centre. You can also examine the differences between centres, the null hypothesis being that such differences are no greater than what one would expect by chance. If the null hypothesis is accepted then you have lost nothing; if the null hypothesis is rejected, then you now know that there are differences between the centres. This fact may be of no interest to you, but it could serve as a hypothesis for investigating the nature and causes of such differences.

This technique, of repeating a simple experiment with groups of subjects which differ in some systematic way, can be extended to other kinds of differences. It can be applied to such quantitative variables as age, length of illness or severity of illness. It can also be applied to qualitative attributes such as pattern of symptoms or type of illness, or different kinds of complications. In each case, the subjects are classified into these groups and then in each group the subjects are randomly allocated to the treatments. It should be obvious by now, that each of these groups form a unit experiment. The allocation to groups should be done beforehand as part of the planning of the experiment but, at a pinch, it could be done at the end of the experiment, if new information suggests that it would be better to do so. Nothing will be lost and something could be gained in this way.

Matched-Pairs Design

When the groups are being sorted out on some quantitative variable, it is necessary to decide how this should be done. If the variable is age, then the subjects could be sorted out into three broad divisions of young, middle aged and old. The groups could be narrowed to decades, twenty to twenty-nine years, thirty to thirty-nine and so on. The age-ranges could be narrowed down to the limit, until finally there are only two subjects of almost exactly the same age in each group, one receiving the one treatment and the second receiving the other. This design goes by the name of 'matched pairs'. In this particular case, the standard methods of statistical analysis can still be used, but it is possible to introduce a simplification by considering the effects of the treatment only in terms of the differences between the results in each pair. Such differences can be analysed in their original quantitative form, but it is also possible to simplify them further by considering merely whether each pair favours one treatment or the other. I shall deal with this in the next lecture.

I must remind you that although I have been talking of a comparison between two treatments, the same principles apply to the simultaneous comparison of three or more treatments, as was shown by the example given previously. In that case, the matched-pairs experiment becomes matched triplets, matched quadruplets, etc.

In a matched-pairs experiment, the difficulty is to decide what is the most important factor on which to make the matching. In the case of an investigation of hypotensive drugs, we might match on blood pressure, age, length of history or rapidity of progress of the illness. That is what I meant when I said in an earlier lecture that sometimes we do not know what are the important factors to be controlled. One way of tackling this problem is to match on all relevant factors but you can see that although it might be easy to match on one factor, it is not likely to be easy to match on two, and to match on three or more is almost impossible.

In reading about research techniques, you may sometimes see reference to the matching of groups. An investigator in education may match classes in order to test different methods of teaching. He does this because a teacher has to teach all the children of a class, and cannot use different methods of teaching for a number of small groups in one class. In such a case, the 'unit' being investigated is the class, not the individual pupil. In the same way, the clinician might compare different regimes in separate wards, and match the wards, but once again, his 'unit' is the ward, not the individual patient. This is an uncommon situation for clinicians, for we usually treat individual patients.

In practice, it is not difficult to match patients on qualitative factors, male and female, sudden or slow onset, Rhesus positive and negative blood-groups, or even at a pinch the A, B, AB and O blood-groups. When it comes to quantitative factors, even if they are divided into a relatively small number of 'levels', the task is almost impossible. There is another way of handling that sort of problem, which I will deal with later.

Cross-Over Design

The best method of matching is to use the same subject for both treatments. In this way, the match is as good as possible; it is not perfect because you cannot give the two treatments simultaneously and people do change in the course of time. This is the method of the 'cross-over' trial. To compare two treatments, we randomly allot our subjects into two groups. Group 1 is given treatment A and group 2 is given treatment B. After a suitable period, the effects of the treatments are measured, and then group 1 is transferred to treatment B, and group 2 to treatment A, and the effects again measured at some appropriate occasion. In this design, which is sometimes called a 'self-controlled' design, not only is the matching as good as possible, but since every subject is used both for the treatment and its control, we have what is effectively twice as many patients. This is the great attraction of this design.

Unfortunately, there are many difficulties in the application of this kind of experiment. Obviously, it must be limited to those conditions and treatments where no permanent effects can be expected from treatment. For example, if we wanted to compare two antibiotics for the treatment of pneumonia, we could not use a cross-over design, because once a patient had recovered it would not be possible to try the other treatment on him. This is a very obvious example, but even in many other conditions, the treatment would have some continued or permanent effect, if it had any at all. A situation very similar to this is where a drug accumulates and is excreted slowly. The cross-over could not be done until all of the first drug had been excreted and this might take a long time. This time would have to be determined first, and an appropriate interval introduced into the procedure. Another difficulty would be that produced by delayed effects of a treatment, i.e. a treatment might initiate some reparative process, which would then proceed even in the absence of the treatment. A common example of this is the effect of even a temporary improvement on the morale of a patient, and his consequent co-operativeness in a difficult or painful therapeutic regime. Finally, one is faced with the natural development of a disease, so that treatment in the early stages may have a very different effect from that in the later stages. I am not trying to decry the cross-over design, but I think that its disadvantages are insufficiently appreciated.

Latin-Square Design

The extension of the cross-over design is the 'latin square' design. Here we compare a number of treatments, say three, giving the subjects all the treatments in such a way that in addition, the three treatments also occur in all the orders, i.e. first, second and third. Table 7.3 makes this quite clear. Labelling the treatments A, B and C; we have the pattern as shown.

TABLE 7.3.   *Latin square design*

	Subject 1	Subject 2	Subject 3	Totals
1st Treatment	A	B	C	For 1st treatment
2nd Treatment	B	C	A	For 2nd treatment
3rd Treatment	C	A	B	For 3rd treatment
Totals	For subject 1	For subject 2	For subject 3	

Latin-square designs can be made for more than three treatments. Of course, we would usually use more than one patient for each of the columns in the diagram, giving a replicated latin-square design. Table 7.3 shows the resemblance of the lay-out of the Latin-square design to a factorial design. Statistical analysis of the difference between columns tells us how much the subjects differ; analysis of the difference between rows tells us what differences there are due to the order of treatments. Finally, we can rearrange the nine results so that treatments A, B and C occupy three separate columns; we can thereby determine the differences between treatments and then eliminate the other two sets of effects.

Sequential Design

In the designs I have described we usually decide beforehand how many subjects we are going to include in the investigation. If they are not all available, we start the experiment as the subjects present themselves, and when we have reached the required number, we stop and analyse the results. Some experience is required to make an estimate of the number required, or we can ask for advice.

It would obviously be a great advantage if we could test our results as we go along, so that we could stop as soon as we had enough cases on which to base a decision. In this way, we could avoid taking too many cases into the trial. There can be no argument against using the minimum number of cases.

The usual method of conducting such a trial is to take a pair of cases (matched appropriately, but this is not necessary), allot them randomly to the two treatments, and then determine the result. If the patient on treatment A does better than the patient on treatment B, then we call the result a ' success ', and if the other way round, we call it a ' failure '. If the two patients do equally well or equally badly, we ignore the result. A diagram can be constructed in such a way that, by plotting the successes and failures on it, we can eventually come to the conclusion that treatment A is significantly better than B or vice versa. An added refinement is that we can also come to the decision that the two treatments do not differ sufficiently to make it worth while going on. See Figure 7.5.

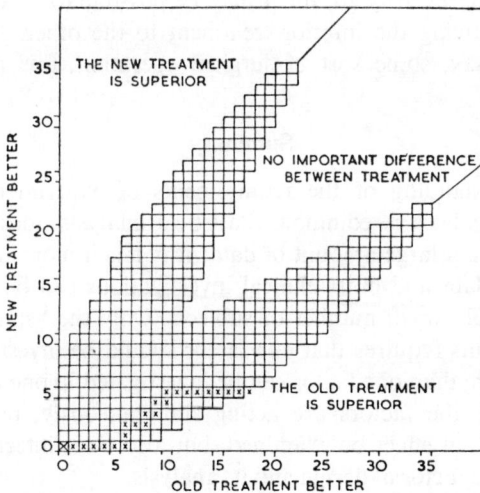

Figure 7.5. Result of test in a sequential trial. Up left-hand side: new treatment better. Along bottom: old treatment better. Reproduced by permission from *British Medical Journal.*

The technique of the sequential trial is a great advance in the design of experiments, but it is not a solution to all problems. There are occasions when it is unsuitable or impracticable. It is at its best when used with matched pairs, and I have already given an account of the difficulties one may meet here. One of the difficulties of matching that I have not mentioned is the need to have the members of the pair available simultaneously. When suitable patients arrive at long intervals this means that the first member of a pair has to be kept waiting until the other one arrives. We cannot toss a coin to allot his treatment and then wait for his companion, because we then know what treatment the newcomer will receive, and this may bias our decision whether to accept the new case into that pair or not. Another limitation of the sequential design is that the time required to record the results of treatment should be less than the time required to collect the cases. For example, we may be making some follow-up inquiry; by the time we start to collect the results from the first few pairs, we may have a long series undergoing observation and waiting for their results. We may soon have enough on which to base a decision, and there are still more cases coming in for final assessment. Under such circumstances, much of the advantages of the sequential design are lost, though not necessarily so, for it may be possible to switch over the patients receiving the inferior treatment to the other. If the treatments are, say, some sort of surgical operation, this may not be possible.

Summary

Misunderstanding of the requirements of experimentation and statistical analysis is common. Statistical analysis does not necessarily require a large amount of data; it is much more important to have good data and most clinical investigations can be carried out on a relatively small number of subjects. Only the ' simple design ' of experiments requires that one factor should be investigated. The effect of more than one factor can be investigated in one experiment, and because the factors are acting simultaneously, not only can their individual effect be examined, but also their interaction. This is done in the factorial design and its analysis.

REFERENCES

HAMILTON, M., HORDERN, A., WALDROP, F. N. & LOFFT, J. (1963). A controlled trial on the value of prochlorperazine, trifluoperazine and intensive group treatment. *British Journal of Psychiatry*, **109**, 510-522.

NEWTON, D. R. L. & TANNER, J. M. (1956). *N*-Acetyl-Para-Aminophenol as an analgesic. *British Medical Journal*, **ii**, 1096-1099.
TRUELOVE, S. C. (1960). Stilboestrol, phenobarbitone and diet in chronic duodenal ulcer. *British Medical Journal*, **ii**, 559-566.

LECTURE EIGHT

Induction: III

In this lecture I leave the problems of experimentation and go on to deal with the problems of induction, i.e. the process by which one draws conclusions from the result of an experiment. To demonstrate this, I will give you some data from a little investigation I carried out a number of years ago. There were 22 patients, diagnosed as suffering from anxiety state, and they were grouped into 11 pairs such that the patients in each pair had approximately the same severity of symptoms. This is known as the 'matched pairs' design. All the patients were interviewed regularly, and given such psychotherapy as seemed appropriate. In addition, one member of the pair received a sedative drug and the other received dummy tablets in the same dosage. At the end of the investigation the symptoms of the patients were assessed to determine which one in each pair had improved more than the other. When I checked what treatment the patients had received I found that in eight pairs the patient who had had the drug had done better that the other member of the pair; in two pairs the patient receiving the drug had done worse and in the last they were approximately equal. Let us ignore the last pair and concentrate on the ten others.

Combinations

The null hypothesis states that the difference between the two groups, the one receiving the drug and the other not and, in particular, the difference between the two patients in each pair, was not due to the effect of the treatment but was due to chance, i.e. in any one pair, one patient was going to do better than the other anyway. Consider any one of the pairs in which the drug did better than the dummy; had I given the treatment in the opposite way then the result would have been worse for the drug. The drug actually did better but it could just as easily have given a worse result. This possible reversal of the result applies to the second pair, the third pair, the fourth and so on. Let us consider all the possible results we could have obtained and write them down for the first four pairs.

88

Figure 8.1

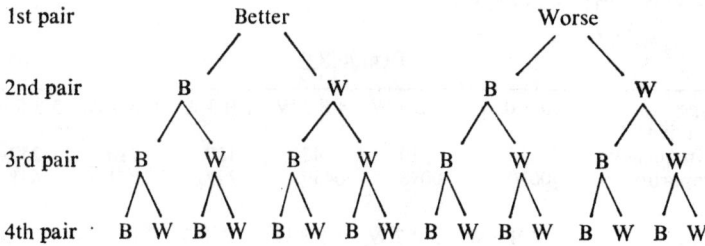

Figure 8.1.

Figure 8.1 enables us to do so easily. The first line of the two triangles shows that the first result may have been either better or worse for the drug. Whatever the first one may have been, the second line shows us that it could have been either better or worse in the second pair and so on. By following every pathway in the two triangles, from the first line to the fourth, we can construct every type of better or worse that could have been obtained. The result is shown in Table 8.1.

TABLE 8.1

B B B B	4, 0	W B B B	3, 1
B B W B	3, 1	W B B W	2, 2
B B B W	3, 1	W B W B	2, 2
B B W W	2, 2	W B W W	1, 3
B W B B	3, 1	W W B B	2, 2
B W B W	2, 2	W W B W	1, 3
B W W B	2, 2	W W W B	1, 3
B W W W	1, 3	W W W W	0, 4

Every one of these was equally likely to occur. Since the four pairs that we are considering do not have any particular order, we need consider only the numbers of better and worse in the total, and these will range from those with four better to those with four worse. If you count them up you will see that the relative proportions will be as follows:

4B,0W	3B,1W	2B,2W	1B,3W	0B,4W
1	4	6	4	1

We can do the same for all ten pairs and I would suggest that you would find it an interesting experience to try it yourself. The results are as follows in Table 8.2.

TABLE 8.2

Type	10 B 0 W	9 B 1 W	8 B 2 W	7 B 3 W	6 B 4 W	5 B 5 W
Relative frequency	1	10	45	120	210	252
Proportion	·0010	·0098	·0439	·1172	·2051	·2461

Type	4 B 6 W	3 B 7 W	2 B 8 W	1 B 9 W	0 B 10 W	Total
Relative frequency	210	120	45	10	1	1024
Proportion	·2051	·1172	·0439	·0098	·0010	1·0001

We could get exactly the same figures by tossing ten coins and counting the number of heads and tails. The number of different combinations is 1024 and the relative frequencies are shown in the table. When these are converted to proportions of the total, they

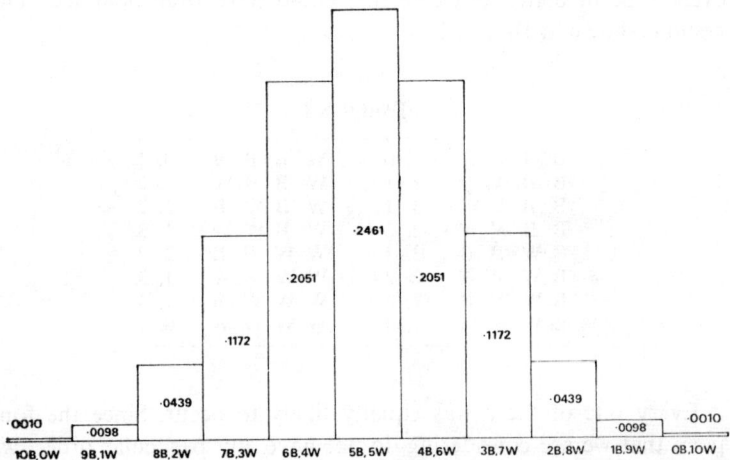

Figure 8.2. Histogram of combinations of order ten.

should add up to one; in fact, owing to errors of rounding, the total is 1·0001, which is near enough. We can show this table in the form of a diagram in which each column has a height proportional to the appropriate figure in the last line of the table. Such a diagram is known as a histogram.

There is one point I have to mention before we study the table and histogram though I cannot go into it in detail. The table gives frequencies, but these are interpreted as probabilities. The probability, or chance, of a given event or result occurring is regarded as equivalent to the frequency with which it will occur if one goes on long enough.

Estimating Probabilities

Consider now all possible combinations of ten results; the probability of getting 10 better and 0 worse is ·001 of the total or, if you prefer it, 0·1 per cent of the total. The probability of getting 8 better and 2 worse is ·0439 or 4·39 per cent. In the histogram, the probability is represented by the height of the column, and since the bases of the column are equal, it is also represented by

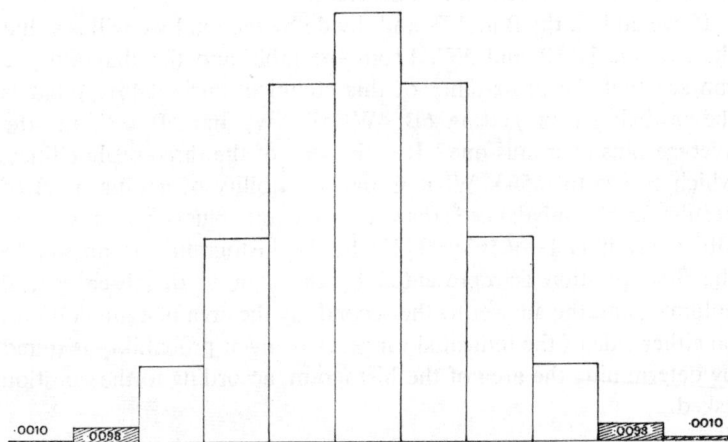

·0010   ·0098   ·0098   ·0010

Figure 8.3. Probability of a disproportion greater than 8:2 of Better and Worse.

the area of the column. What is the probability of getting 5 better and 5 worse? From the table it is ·2461. What is the probability of not getting 5 better and 5 worse? Obviously, it is 1 − ·2461, and this comes to ·7539. Notice that although the commonest result gives equal numbers of better and worse, the probability of not getting it is about three times as much as the probability of getting it. If you think it over you will see that this result will help explain to you the phenomenon which always seems queer when one first meets it. The typical case of a disease is usually the commonest one, and yet it is surprising that one sees it only relatively infrequently. Atypical cases are usually much commoner than typical ones.

What is the probability of getting 1 worse and 9 better? It is ·0098. What is the probability of getting 0 worse and 10 better? It is ·001. What is the probability of getting either one or none worse in the ten? Obviously, it is the sum of the two, which is ·0108. In the histogram, it is the area of the first two columns on the left. This question is equivalent to asking the probability of getting 9 or more better. What is the probability of getting a disproportion between better and worse greater than 8:2? It is the probability of getting more than 8 better added to the probability of getting more than 8 worse, and this comes to ·0216. In the histogram, it is represented by the sum of the areas of the two end columns on the left and on the right.

If we add all the B and W and divide by the total we will see that the average is 5B and 5W. From the table and the diagram, we can see that the probability of this combination is ·2461. What is the probability of getting 6B 4W, 5B 5W, and 4B 6W, i.e. the average plus or minus one? It is the sum of the three probabilities, which comes to ·6563. What is the probability of getting a set of results more unbalanced than the average plus or minus one? Obviously it is $1 - ·6563 = ·3437$. In the histogram, the answer to the first question is represented by the area of the three central columns, and the answer to the second, by the area of eight columns on either side of the indicated range. Any given probability is found by determining the area of the histogram, according to the question asked.

Interpreting the Results

We found that the patients who received the drug did better than those who didn't in the proportion of 8:2. What is the probability that we could have got a result as good as this or better? It is the sum of the areas of the three left hand columns and comes to ·0547. Let us be clear what this signifies. If we assume that the null hypothesis is true, i.e. that the drug has no effect, then, if the experiment were to be repeated a very large number of times, we would find that in $5\frac{1}{2}$ per cent of the experiments we would have obtained a result as good as this or better in favour of the drug.

In statistical terms, the results are significant at the $5\frac{1}{2}$ per cent level. Suppose we had been comparing two different drugs, there would then have been no reason for assuming that one was better than the other and we would have had to consider simply the differences between them, i.e. not only that the first drug was better than the second, but also the second was better than the first. We would have had to take into account the right-hand columns as well as the left-hand columns. This would give us a statistical significance at the 11 per cent level. The former test of significance is known as the one-tailed and the latter as the two-tailed test, for obvious reasons.

In the experiment just described, the subject in each pair who had received the drug was described as having been better or worse than the control subject. How much better or worse was not mentioned (though the original data did give this). Classifying results in this way into crude categories loses a great deal of information, though in some cases the data naturally fall into two classes. This applies obviously to such indices as death rates, discharge rates, or even the need to carry out a surgical operation or not. In most clinical research, the data consists of measurements on some sort of scale. The advantages of using such quantitative measures (variables) is so great that researchers often go to great lengths to convert data into quantitative form, although they are primarily in the form of distinct categories. The opposite procedure is sometimes used because of its great convenience and despite the loss of information it entails. For example, age will be converted into young, middle aged, and old; height may be categorized into short, average, and tall; and even improvement may be dichotomized into a need to continue with supervision or not.

Descriptive Statistics

If we record a thousand systolic blood pressures, we find it is impossible to comprehend these thousand figures as such. Some way must be found to compress the information so that it can be grasped. The simplest way is to count how many times each value of the measurement occurs and this gives us a 'frequency distribution'. A 'distribution' implies a scattering around some sort of centre and this introduces us to two of the basic concepts in statistical theory: the measure of central tendency and the measure of scatter or variability. When we plot a frequency distribution as a histogram, we can intuitively see what is meant by the ' shape ' of a frequency distribution. This is a third basic concept. The shape of a distribution can be defined in algebraic terms quite rigorously but I shall not go into it here.

In common speech, the word average is used to describe the central tendency of a group, but the statistician distinguishes between three kinds. The commonest is the mean, which is obtained by adding a set of figures and dividing by the number of figures. The mean of a group is an abstract notion and can be calculated to a degree of accuracy far greater than any of the individual constituent measurements. Furthermore, the mean may not have a real existence. For example, it is possible to calculate the mean of a height of a group of men without any one man having that particular height. Ignorance of this point is sometimes deliberate; some people seem to derive mild amusement from the statement that the average family has, say, 2·4 children and ·05 divorces.

There is another measure of central tendency, or average, which avoids this difficulty. In a given frequency distribution, the measure which has the highest frequency (occurs most commonly) is the mode. It will help you to remember the definition of the term if you realize that in common speech, mode has a meaning equivalent to fashion. Using our example once again, the modal family will have two children and no divorces. An important property of the mean is that there can be only one mean of a group but this is not true of the mode. If we look at the histogram of a frequency distribution we may see that sometimes it does not have one hump somewhere between the two ends but two or more, in which case the frequency distribution is bimodal, trimodal and so on.

The third measure of central tendency is the median and this means simply the middle. If you arrange a set of measurements into ascending or descending order, then the median is the middle one. There may be several modes, there is only one mean but unfortunately there is sometimes no median. If the number of measurements is even, then the middle lies between the two of the measurements; it is customary then to give the median as being the means of these two adjacent measures.

Variability

Consider the following set of twenty numbers, which we may regard as the age of as many patients :

Series A

31,33,35,38,38, 41,43,47,47,47, 51,54,54,58,58, 61,64,64,67,69.

Their mean is 50 and they are so distributed that 10 are below the mean and 10 above, i.e. the distribution is symmetrical. Suppose these numbers were written on slips of paper, put into a box, and one drawn at random. The probability of drawing a number below 50 is a half, or ·5. If we put the number back and draw another, the probability that the second will be below the mean is also ·5. The probability that both will be below the mean is ·5 × ·5, or ·25. The probability that a third drawn in the same way will be below the mean is also a half, and the probability that all three will be below the mean is ·125.

In the same way, we can see that the probability of drawing a number below 45 is 7/20 or ·35. The probability of drawing two numbers below 45 is 7/20 × 7/20, or ·1225, and of drawing three below 45 is ·0429.

Let us now look at the next series of numbers:

Series B

40,41,43,43,43, 46,46,47,47,49, 51,53,53,53,55, 56,56,59,59,60.

If we draw numbers from this series in the same way as before, the probability of drawing one below the mean is ·5, or drawing two is ·25 and of three is ·125. This is the same as in series A. The probability of drawing a number less than 45 is 5/20 or ·25, of drawing two is ·0625 and of three is ·0156. These last three probabilities are less than those from series A. The difference between the two series is obviously due to the differences in variability, or scatter, of the two series.

Measuring Scatter (or Variation)

The simplest way of measuring scatter is to give the range of the figures. Although both series have a mean of 50, series A runs from 31 to 69, or 39 points, and series B runs from 40 to 60, or 20 points. In other words, we can say that in series A the highest figure is 38 points above the lowest, and in series B it is 20. This statement is equivalent to reckoning the lowest figure as our starting point, counting it as zero, and measuring the other figures as ' deviations ' from the lowest point.

Another way is to reckon the figures as deviations from the

mean, so that series A would have a range of -19 to $+19$, and series B of -10 to $+10$.

There are two obvious reasons why the range is unsatisfactory as a measure of scatter in a series of numbers or measurements. The first is that it is extremely unstable. Taking these figures as the ages of a series of patients, the next patient might be 80 years old, which would about double the range in series B. When we compare this with the effect on the mean, which would increase by a mere four points almost, we can see what is meant by the instability of the range and the stability of the mean. The second reason why the range is unsatisfactory is that it takes into account only the extreme figures, and ignores the intermediate ones. The range would be the same whether most of the figures clustered near one point or were evenly distributed. A good measure of scatter should take into account all the figures, in the same way as does the mean.

At first glance, it would seem that a simple way of doing this would be to take all the figures as deviations from the mean and average them. But, of course, the total of the deviations from the mean comes to zero. That is one way of defining the mean: it is that point from which the deviations on either side balance out. One way of dealing with this difficulty is to ignore the pluses and minuses when averaging the deviations. This figure is known as the average deviation. It has the advantage of being simple and easy to understand, but this is its only merit.

The statistician tackles the problem in a different way. He takes the measures as deviations from the mean, and gets rid of the difficulty with the signs by squaring the deviations. Whether the deviations are positive or negative, the squared deviations are all positive, and it is then simple to sum them and take the average. This average of the squared deviations from the mean is known as variance. (As a matter of interest, the sum of the squared deviations is sometimes referred to as the deviance.) The variance has many important properties which make it the centre of interest in statistical analysis, but it has one disadvantage: it is the wrong unit. In the examples taken, the deviations are so many years above or below the mean; the squared deviations and the variance are ' squared years ', a quantity which has no physical meaning. If we consider a group of heights, the variance will be measured in terms of square centimetres, and although this has a physical meaning, it is the wrong unit when we are considering the scatter of a set of heights. This difficulty is easily solved by taking the square root of the variance, which restores the original unit. The square root of the variance is known as the standard deviation, and this too has many important properties.

Samples from a Population

Suppose we have collected a large set of figures, which may be measurements or scores. The greater the scatter of the numbers is, then the greater is the variance and standard deviation. We now select randomly a small group of the scores, i.e. we take a random 'sample' from the 'population' of numbers. Conceivably, they could all be identical but this is obviously very unlikely. Usually, they will differ and, if the scatter of the original population is large, then we would expect the scores in our sample to be widely scattered, and vice versa. The variance and standard deviation of our sample are likely to be related to the corresponding figures of the parent population. The same will be true of a second sample. In general, we would expect the two samples to differ; not only will their variance differ but, what is more to the point, their means will differ. I am sure that you will have little difficulty in seeing that if the variance of the original population is large then the means are likely to differ by a great amount, and vice versa.

TABLE 8.3

Improvement Scores in Three Groups of 21 Cases

1. PCP			2. TFP			3. PLAC		
−2	10	21	0	13	22	−20	5	19
−1	10	22	6	15	28	−11	7	19
−1	11	23	8	16	29	−8	7	20
4	13	24	9	18	31	−7	9	25
6	18	29	9	18	32	−	13	25
6	19	32	11	20	34	−	14	26
7	21	38	12	21	49	4	18	31

The implications of this can best be explained by considering an actual example. Table 8.3 contains three sets of figures. Each figure is a score which represents the amount of improvement in the symptoms of a patient (worsening if the number is negative). The data are obtained from an investigation in which I participated a number of years ago. The patients' symptoms were assessed and they were then given treatment. After a suitable interval their symptoms were assessed again. The improvement was measured by the difference between the two scores. Group PCP received one drug, group TFP received the second drug and group P received a dummy or placebo. For your convenience, the figures have been arranged in ascending order. Figure 8.4 gives the same information as the table but in a way which is easy to grasp. The means of the two drug treated groups are higher than the group given placebo, i.e. they show a greater improvement on the average. The null hypo-

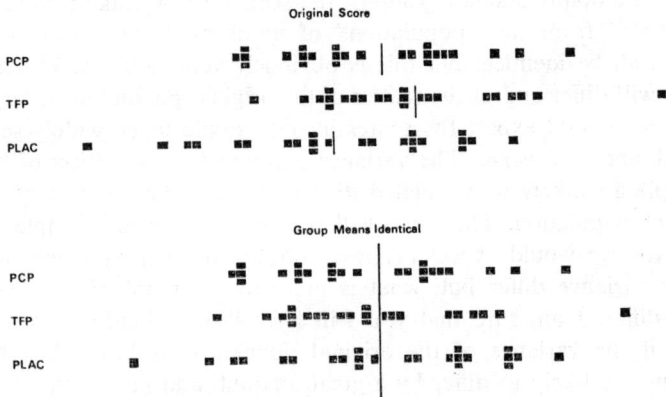

Figure 8.4. Improvement scores of three groups.

thesis is that the differences between the groups, and especially the differences between the means of the groups, is due to chance: the accident of allocation of the patients to the different treatments. Put in another way, the differences between the groups are no greater than what we would expect by taking three samples randomly from a ' population '. If we were to calculate the probability of obtaining such differences and we then found it sufficiently small, we would reject the null hypothesis. We would say that we preferred to believe that findings are not a chance result, but that the differences between the means of the groups is due to the effects of the active treatments.

We have first to find some way of estimating the variance of the population and then use this for calculating the probability. I shall explain in detail how this is done in due course but I shall indicate the general principle now. If you look at the figure and consider the three groups as one, it is obvious that the scatter of the total is greater than the scatter of the individual group. Our positive hypothesis states that the active drugs have increased the amount of improvement in the patients receiving them and therefore, in the diagram, have shifted them further to the right than they would otherwise have been. This has the effect of increasing the scatter of the total. Speaking more precisely, the effects of the drugs have been to increase the variance of the total number of cases. If the drugs had no effect, then groups PCP and TFP would be located further to the left and the total variance would be that much less. If we shift the groups so that their means coincide, as shown in Figure 8.4, we can see that the scatter is reduced.* we can now calculate the variance and compare it with the original variance. The difference between the two is obviously due to the differences between the means of the three groups, since the relative positions of each patient in each group is unchanged. We now have two explanations for the discrepancy between these two variances: the positive hypothesis states that it is due to the effects of the drugs and the null hypothesis states that it is due to chance.

Summary

A frequency distribution can be represented visually in the form of a histogram, which has the property that probabilities can be shown as appropriately defined areas. Two fundamental notions in statistical theory are those of central tendency and dispersion or scatter. The former is indicated by the mean, mode and median; the latter by variance and standard deviation. The effects of treatments and other factors can be considered in terms of their influence on variance.

REFERENCE

HAMILTON, A., HORDERN, A., WALDROP, F. N. & LOFFT, J. (1963). *British Journal of Psychiatry*, **109**, 510-522.

* You may think that the reduction is trivial, but I assure you that it is statistically significant. Tests of statistical significance are really quite sensitive!

Analysis of Variance

In the previous lecture I gave you a brief introduction to some of the fundamental ideas of statistics and, to illustrate them, I gave a specific example. This consisted of three sets of data, being the results of treatment of three groups of patients. I tried to give you some indication of how the probability of the null hypothesis could be calculated. By now, you will realize that such probability will be estimated in terms of an area under a curve. Since the areas of this curve have already been calculated, and are to be found in appropriate tables, it would be quite feasible and very simple to show the steps of the calculation and to show you how to look up the results in the table. Since these lectures are intended to give some understanding of the underlying principles rather than to describe a set of routine procedures which could be carried out quite mechanically and without thinking, I shall now go on to consider some basic theory.

Theory of Variation (Errors)

It is obvious that individuals differ, and sometimes they can differ considerably. Let us consider a specific variable, which simply means a particular attribute or characteristic that is quantitatively different in different individuals, or on different occasions, when it is measured. When we think about the differences between individuals on such measures as height, weight, blood-pressure, metabolic rate, and even such things as cheerfulness or irritability, we can recognize that these differences are sometimes due to causes or factors which give rise to great differences, for example, sex, age, the presence of disease, and so on. Other causes produce only small differences, and in most cases, we recognize that there are likely to be many such, of which we know nothing or very little. Let us ignore the causes of major differences (which we handle in our investigations by using them as categories of classification), and consider only the factors which give rise to small differences.

These factors will either be independent or not. When they are dependent, i.e. when the occurrence of one tends to produce the

100

occurrence of another, we may regard these factors as one, to the extent that they occur together and tend to produce the same sort of effect, and as separate and independent to the extent that they do not. When these linked factors are sufficient to give rise to a major effect, they can be recognized and dealt with in the usual way. We are then left with a group of factors producing minor effects, and independent of each other in their action.

These factors can have only one effect on the variable: by their presence or absence they will tend to increase the variable or decrease it. If they all act in one direction, they will increase the variable by a large amount, and if in the opposite direction, they will decrease it by a large amount. If they act in the opposite directions they will tend to cancel out each other. If we take these presuppositions as a basis for theoretical development, it can be shown that large effects will tend to occur infrequently and small ones will tend to occur frequently. If we plot the distribution of our measures in the population assuming it to be indefinitely large, we will obtain a bell-shaped curve. Such a distribution is known as a Gaussian or ' normal ' distribution. (This does not mean that other types of distribution are ' abnormal '!)

If we turn now to the histogram in Figure 8.2, we see that it is similar to the Gaussian distribution, but that the top of the strips form a staircase instead of a smooth curve. It can be shown that as the number of sub-divisions (which determine the number of strips in the histogram) increases indefinitely, the figure tends to look more and more like the Gaussian distribution.

The Gaussian (' Normal ') Distribution

The Gaussian distribution has many important properties. One of the most interesting, and most valuable, arises from the fact that if we take a sample from a population by random selection (which means that each individual has an equal chance of being taken) and calculate its mean; if then we take many such samples, all of the same size, calculate the mean of each and then plot the distribution of the means, this distribution will be Gaussian, or close to it, whatever may have been the distribution of measures in the population. The greater the size of the samples, the nearer will be the distribution of their means to the Gaussian form. Examination of Table 4.1 will serve to illustrate this, especially if you imagine or draw the histogram. Take note that each of the ten values occurs only once, or alternatively, the values occur with equal frequency. Of course the size of the sample was only five cases, and the samples were drawn from a 'population' of only ten figures. Had the population been much larger and the sample size a little larger, the distribution curve would have been extremely close to the Gaussian (normal). Of course, if the original distribution is Gaussian, the distribution of the means of samples will be Gaussian too.

A second important property of the Gaussian distribution concerns its variance. Suppose we have a large 'population' of measures which have a Gaussian distribution. The variance of the distribution we shall call V. We then select randomly a sample of ten measures and calculate the mean of this sample. We repeat this a very large number of times. We then have a large number of such means and we can plot their distribution and calculate its variance. What is the relation between the latter variance and the former? The answer has a delightful simplicity: it is one tenth. Had we taken samples of 20, then the variance of the means of such samples would have been one twentieth of the variance of the population. In general terms, the variance of the distributions of means of samples of a given size is inversely proportional to the size of the samples. (This may be difficult to grasp at first, but it is worthwhile re-reading until you have it.)

A Gaussian distribution is based upon the theoretical notion of an infinite population. Obviously, since it is infinite, there is no way of calculating its mean and variance. All we can do is to take samples from the population, calculate their means and standard deviation and use these as estimates of the true mean and variance. The figures we calculate are known as statistics, and they are estimates of the true figures which are called parameters. A statistic is a figure calculated from a sample and it varies from one sample to another but a parameter is a constant.

A third important property of the Gaussian distribution is that the mean and variance are independent. The corresponding statistics are also independent: for example, if the mean of a sample is larger than the population mean, the variance of the sample could be smaller or greater than the population variance and either way would happen equally often in the long run. The same would apply if the mean of the sample were smaller than the mean of the population. This can be proved mathematically but it can be seen intuitively from the fact that the variance is calculated by taking deviations from the mean. In other words, whatever the sample mean may be, it is always reckoned as zero. Whether the mean of your sample be too low or too high it is still counted as zero and the variance calculated from it.

An important property of variances is that when independent they are additive. Let me explain this by an example. We take a sample of ten figures and calculate its mean. We take a second sample and calculate its mean. In general, these two means will differ. We subtract one from the other and note the difference. We repeat this a large number of times: taking two samples and subtracting their means. We then have a large number of such differences. They have a distribution and it in its turn has a variance. What is the size of this variance of difference between means? The answer is simple, it is the sum of the variance of the means. The variance of the means is $V/10$ and the variance of the differences between the means is $V/10+V/10=V/5$. This is true even if the samples are of different size. Suppose that in each pair of samples, one contains five figures and the other ten. The variance of the means of the one will be $V/5$ and of the other $V/10$. The variance of the differences between these means will be $V/5+V/10$ $=3V/10$.

What has all this to do with drawing conclusions from the results of experiments? Two more steps, and you will see. You will remember that the square root of the variance is the standard deviation. In the Gaussian distribution, the standard deviation can be found graphically by locating the point where the curve changes from convex to concave. At this point, the curve is 'straight' and the tangent (the line which just touches the curve and marks its slope) cuts the curve. If we take our measures as deviations from the mean, i.e. if, when plotting the curve, we take the mean as zero, so that the curve lies symmetrically on either side of the ordinate (y axis), then the height of the curve at any given point, as a proportion of the greatest height, is determined by the distance of that point from the mean (along the X axis) when given in terms of the standard deviation. We can draw this line and measure it but this is not necessary as its height has already been calculated and can be found by looking up the table of the Gaussian distribution. The area under the curve is cut into two parts by this line and the proportion of the sizes of these two areas has also been calculated.

The next step is easy, once you see it. Just as in the histogram, we could determine probabilities by measuring areas, so we can do the same in the Gaussian distribution. The probability of obtaining, by random selection, a measure greater than a given size is equivalent to finding the area on the right of the curve which is beyond the point which marks that given measure. Thus, it is easy to determine the probability of obtaining more than one standard deviation above the mean, or more than two standard deviations above

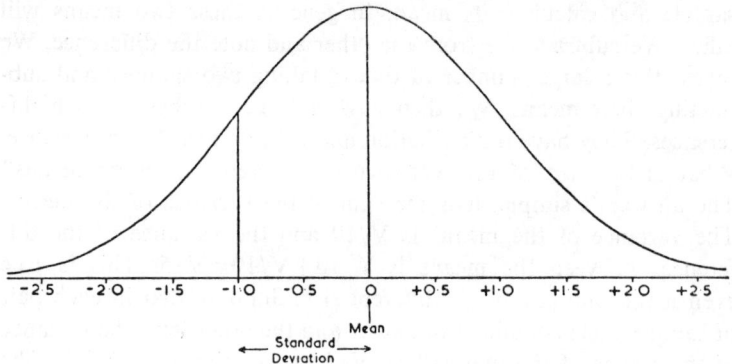

Figure 9.1. The Gaussian (normal) distribution.

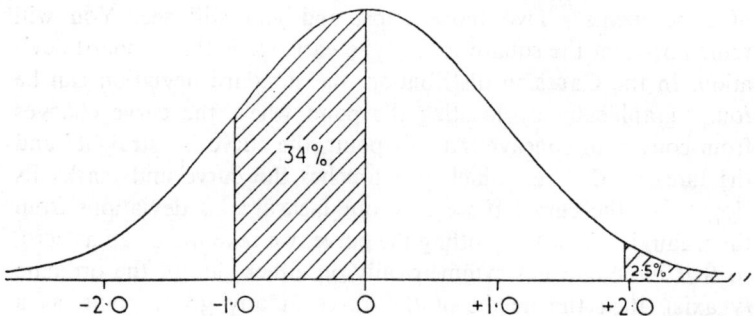

Figure 9.2. Probabilities as areas.

the mean. If we consider the figures less than the mean, we take the area to the left of the mean corresponding to those on the right. If we want to determine the probability of obtaining a measure within one standard deviation of the mean, we measure the appropriate area in the centre of the curve. As they have already been calculated, we can save ourselves the trouble of making these measurements by looking them up in the tables.

Sample and Population

The variance of a ' population ' of figures is obtained by taking each figure as a deviation from the mean, i.e. subtracting the mean from the figure, then squaring the deviations, adding them and taking the average. In practice, however many subjects we take, we always regard them as a sample from a more general population. We cannot therefore subtract the population mean from each figure in order to obtain the deviation, because the population mean is unknown. All we have is the mean of the sample before us. The use of the sample mean for calculating the variance has peculiar implications which are of fundamental importance.

A random sample from a population is defined as being one in which each member of the population has an equal chance of being taken into the sample and this choice of each member is independent of the others. This means that when a particular individual is chosen, it makes no difference to the chances of the others. Let us consider the following five figures as a random sample selected from a population of figures. They are 12, 8, 5, 14 and 11. The total comes to 50 and the mean is 10. Knowing that the mean of the sample is 10, we can rewrite these figures as deviations from the mean: +2, −2, −5, +4, +1. The sum of these five deviations should come to zero and if you check them you will see that it does. Imagine now that these five numbers are on five slips of paper put into a box, shaken about and then picked out unseen one by one. When we pick out the first, we do not know what it is until we look at it. The same applies to the second, third and fourth, but before we pick out the fifth we know already what it will be. Since we know the total of the first four numbers the fifth can have only one possible value. Only four of the figures in the sample are independent since they determine the fifth, and this applies to any four. In technical terms, when we calculate the mean from a sample, we decrease its *degrees of freedom* by one and if the sample contains n figures then the degrees of freedom are n−1.

If we are interested in the variance of a given set of figures only, then we divide the sum of squared deviations from the mean (the deviance) by the number of figures in the group. But if we want to use our samples in order to estimate the variance of the population, we divide the deviance by the degrees of freedom. It is not difficult to prove why this should be so and many elementary textbooks on statistics give the proof. Strictly speaking, using the degrees of freedom as the divisor gives an unbiased estimate of the variance of the population, i.e. in the long run these estimates tend more and more to the correct figure.

The Gaussian distribution is based on a population of infinite size and therefore it has an infinite number of degrees of freedom. If the curve is calculated or drawn, with the assumption that the degrees of freedom are finite, the shape of the curve is somewhat different. The Gaussian distribution is in fact the last of a family of curves, the first being based on one degree of freedom, the second on two degrees of freedom and so on. These curves have already been calculated, not all (of course!) but enough for practical purposes. After about a hundred degrees of freedom or so, the curve is almost identical with the Gaussian curve based on its infinite degrees of freedom. When therefore we wish to determine any probability in the area under a curve, we must use that one which is based on the current number of degrees of freedom or use the appropriate section of the table.

Estimating Population Variance

We have to estimate the variance of the population from our three sets of figures in the example, and we can do this in different ways. We can take the 63 figures and calculate the variance from

TABLE 9.1

Variance of Population from Means

Group	Means	Deviations	Squared deviations
1. PCP	14·761905	·412699	·170320
2. TFP	19·095238	4·746032	22·524820
3. PLAC	9·190476	−5·158730	26·612495
Total	43·047619	·000001	49·307635

General Mean = 43·047619/3   = 14·349206
No. of cases in groups   = 21
Degrees of freedom between groups = 3−1 = 2

Variance of Means = Deviance/d.f.
          = 49·307635/2
          = 24·653818
Variance of population = Variance of means ×
          Size of groups
          = 517·7302

all of them. We add them up and obtain a total and divide this by 63 to give the general mean. We subtract this mean from each figure and obtain the deviations from the mean; we then square these deviations, sum the squares and divide by 62, the degrees of freedom. This is an extremely laborious way of making the calculation and, in practice, a short-cut method is always used. I shall show you this later.

The variance of a population can also be estimated from the variance of means of samples taken from that population. We have three samples and therefore three sample means and we can estimate the variance of the population from them.

Table 9.1 gives the three means and the general mean. The three deviations from the general mean are then shown. These are squared and summed, giving the deviance. There are three means, so the degrees of freedom are two. Dividing the deviance by two gives the variance of the means. You will remember that the variance of means of samples is inversely proportional to the size of the samples. The samples have 21 cases and therefore the variance of the population is 21 times the variance of the means and this is the final figure in the table.

Finally, we can estimate the variance of the population from each sample. For each one, we have first to calculate the deviance or, as it is often known, the corrected sum of squares. Table 9·2 shows how this is done. The right half shows the formal way and the left half is the short-cut method. The table is self-explanatory. You can see that the formal method is not only much longer, but the calculation of the mean and the deviations from the mean have to be carried to a very large number of significant figures to guarantee accuracy. In the short method only the last step requires many significant figures. The deviance of group 1 (PCP) comes to 2521·8095, and although I have not shown the calculations, the deviance from group 2 (TFP) comes to 2659·8095 and the deviance for group 3 (PLAC) comes to 3783·2381. From each group we can estimate the variance of the population by dividing its deviance by the number of degrees of freedom, 20. We will have a better estimate by taking the average of the three groups. This is done by summing the deviances and dividing by the sum of the degrees of freedom, 60. In symbolic form, if n_1, n_2 and n_3 are the number of subjects in the three groups, and D_1, D_2 and D_3 are the corresponding deviances, then what we calculate is $(D_1 + D_2 + D_3)/(n_1 + n_2 + n_3 - 3)$. This comes to 149·4143.

TABLE 9.2

Calculation of Deviance for Group 1 (PCP)

Short-cut method		Formal Method		
Scores	Squares	Scores	Deviations	Squared deviations
−2	4	−2	− 16·761905	280·961459
24	576	24	9·238095	85·342399
10	100	10	−4·761905	22·675739
18	324	18	3·238095	10·485259
4	16	4	− 10·761905	115.818599
22	484	22	7·238095	52·390019
29	841	29	14·238095	202·723349
7	49	7	−7·761905	60·247169
38	1,444	38	23·238095	540·009059
19	361	19	4·238095	17·961449
−1	1	−1	− 15·761905	248·437649
21	441	21	6·238095	38·913829
32	1,024	32	17·238095	297·151919
13	169	13	−1·761905	3·104309
−1	1	−1	− 15·761905	248·437649
23	529	23	8·238095	67·866209
6	36	6	−8·761905	76·770979
10	100	10	−4·761905	22·675739
11	121	11	−3·761905	14·151929
6	36	6	−8·761905	76·770979
21	441	21	6·238095	38·913829
Totals 310	7,098	310	−·000005	2521·809519 ⎱

$$7098 - (310 \times 310)/21 = 7098 - 4576\cdot190476 = 2521\cdot809524$$

This may seem an odd way of doing it. If one wants to take an average why not take the three variances and divide by three, i.e $(V_1 + V_2 + V_3)/3$? Indeed, if you do it that way the answer comes out the same and I would urge you to try it out. The reason for summing the deviances and dividing them by the summed degrees of freedom is because this is a general way, applicable when the groups are of different size. If you want to obtain a general mean from means derived from samples of different sizes, you must first weight these means with the sample size. This is a complicated way of explaining something which is best illustrated with an example. In the following two samples, the first consists of two figures 4 and 6 and the second of six figures 4, 5, 6, 7, 9, and 11. The mean of the first group is $(4+6)/2=5$. The mean of the second group is $42/6=7$. The average of these two means comes to 6, but this is not the mean of the total for if you add up all the figures the mean comes to $52/8=6\frac{1}{2}$. To obtain the correct general mean from the two means each one must be weighted, i.e. multiplied by, the number of figures from which the mean is derived. This comes to $(2\times5+6\times7)/8=52/8=6\frac{1}{2}$.

The variance of the population derived in this way comes to 149·4143. It is known, for obvious reasons, as the 'within-groups' variance. It is much smaller than the estimate of the population variance obtained from the means of the groups, this latter estimate being known as the 'between-groups' variance. The between-groups variance is so much larger than the within-groups variance because, according to our hypothesis, the drug-treated groups have improved much more than the placebo-treated group. This has shifted their means far away from the mean of the placebo-treated group. Alternatively, the null hypothesis says that the increased means of the drug-treated groups are a chance result. The variance estimated from the total number of cases comes to 164·2954 and it is larger than the within-groups variance because of the wide disparity between the means. In general terms, the scatter of the total has been increased over the scatter within the groups because of the scatter between the groups. As you will see, this is an exact description if we consider deviances.

We have obtained two estimates of the variance of the population, 517·7302 and 149·4143. The former is almost three and a half times the latter. More accurately, this ratio, which is known as the F ratio, comes to 3·47. We can determine the probability of obtaining such a result by looking up the tables, taking into account that the numerator of this number is derived from 2 degrees of freedom and the denominator from 60. The table shows that this probability is less than 0·05. This means that if we repeated this experiment often enough we would obtain a ratio as large as 3·47 or larger, not quite 5 times in a 100, if the treatments did not differ in their effects, i.e. if the three groups were merely random samples from the same population.

Layout of Calculation

The analysis of variance may appear to be a very complicated procedure, but this is only because the calculation has been obscured by the need to explain the underlying principles. The procedure is really remarkably simple and to demonstrate this I have laid out the calculation in Table 9.3. It will pay you to study it carefully.

TABLE 9.3

Layout of Statistical Analysis

| | Three Groups | | | |
	Group PCP	Group TFP	Group PLAC	Total
No. of cases	21	21	21	63
Total score	310	401	193	904
Crude sum of squares	7,098	10,317	5,557	22,972
Deviance	$7,098 - 310^2/21$	$10,317 - 401^2/21$	$5,557 - 193^2/21$	
	$= 2,521 \cdot 8095$	$= 2,659 \cdot 8095$	$= 3,783 \cdot 2381$	
Variance = dev./d.f.	126·0905	132·9905	189·1619	
Means	14·7619	19·0952	9·1905	

Sum of squares for

Total	$22,972 - 904^2/63 =$	10,000·3175
Between groups	$310^2/21 + 401^2/21 + 193^2/21 - 904^2/63 =$	1,035·4604
Within groups	$10,000 \cdot 3175 - 1,035 \cdot 4604$	8,964·8571
Check	$2,521 \cdot 8095 + 2,659 \cdot 8095 + 3,783 \cdot 2381 =$	8964·8571

Analysis of variance

Source	df.	Sum of squares	Mean squares	F	P
Between groups	2	1,035·4604	517·7302	3·47	$< \cdot 05$
Within groups	60	8,964·8571	149·4143		
Total	62	10,000·3175			

The first step in the calculation of analysis of variance is to calculate the sums of scores and sums of squares of scores separately for each group. This is the most laborious part of the calculation and has to be done carefully and then checked. The work will be very much easier if you have access to a calculating machine with a ' squaring lock ', i.e. one which will calculate the square of a number and sum the numbers and their squares as you go along. If you can do this, you first add up all the figures in each group to produce the total score. You then repeat this, at the same time calculating sums of squares. If at the end the total score is the same as the one you already have, you can be sure that the sum of squares is correct. These figures are then entered into your sheet as shown. There are three columns of figures for the three groups and a fourth for the totals. The first entry is the number of cases, which in this case is the same for all three groups but need not necessarily be so. The next row gives the total scores for each of the three groups and the grand total and then finally comes the crude sum of squares. For each group we then calculate the deviance, i.e. the sums of squares of deviations from the mean. This is shown, using the short-cut formula, in the next row. The row below shows the three variances, obtained by dividing the deviances by the appropriate number of degrees of freedom, i.e. one less than the number of cases on the group. Finally, for your convenience the next line shows the mean of each group. If you want to calculate the overall mean of all the cases, this should not be entered in the fourth column which is always a total of the other three columns.

All the preliminary calculations for the analysis of variance have now been completed and you are now in a position to check whether the increases in the means from one group to the next are accompanied by increases in the variance. In this particular case it can be seen that this is not so. To calculate the sum of squares for total, i.e. the deviance of all the figures considered as one group, you take the crude sum of squares and subtract from it a ' correcting factor '. This is the grand total, squared and then divided by the number of cases. The calculation of the sum of squares between groups is shown in the next line. In each group, the total is taken, squared and then divided by the number of cases in that group. These are all added together and the correcting factor subtracted. It may be worth your while to calculate the correcting factor separately so as to avoid having to do it each time. Finally, the sum of squares within groups is then obtained by subtracting the sum of squares between groups from the sum of squares for total. To check the accuracy of your calculations, you sum the three deviances obtained above and they should be equal to the figure you have just calculated, as shown in the table. In practice, you would have summed them already. The last step is to calculate the F ratio and look up the probability in the tables.

Finally, the analysis of variance is laid out formally as shown at the bottom of Table 9.3. The degrees of freedom for total are the number of cases less one, $63-1=62$; the degrees of freedom between groups is the number of groups less one, $3-1=2$. The within groups degrees of freedom is most easily obtained by subtraction $62-2=60$. The sums of squares are written in the column as shown and it will be seen that the between-groups and within-groups sums of squares together equal the total. You will now understand more clearly what I meant when I said that the ' variability ' of the total set of figures can be divided into two parts: that within each group and that due to the differences between groups. The mean squares are obtained by dividing the sum of squares by their appropriate degrees of freedom. The within-groups mean square is an estimate of the variance of the population, derived from all the data but independent of the differences between the means of the groups. It is often referred to as the 'error variance'. The between-groups mean squares, or between-groups variance, is then divided by the error variance to give the F ratio. The last figure, the probability of the null hypothesis, is obtained by looking up the tables of the F ratio with two degrees of freedom for the numerator and sixty degrees of freedom for the denominator.

Summary

This lecture has been concerned with the theory of errors (variation) and the Gaussian (normal) distribution. The parameters of this distribution are the mean and standard deviation. The square of the latter is the variance. Whatever the distribution of a population of figures, the means of samples tend to have a Gaussian distribution. The probability of the null hypothesis, which is concerned with the differences between means, is obtained from estimating the area under the curve of the normal distribution. More precisely, from a similar curve, the exact shape of which is determined by the degree of freedom. This is the basis for the statistical test known as the analysis of variance.

Practical Problems in Experiments

It would be logical to continue with the subject of the design of experiments and their statistical analysis, but the previous lectures have been difficult, so instead I shall return to the subject of experimentation and consider in detail certain practical aspects.

The Trial Experiment

Before an experiment is started it is well to do a preliminary or trial experiment. It is only in this way that one has an opportunity of seeing the practical difficulties that can appear. In clinical research, the preliminary trial is largely a test of what one might call the administrative procedures, but sometimes the work requires more than plain observation of patients, one will be using apparatus. In such cases, a preliminary trial is absolutely necessary to ensure that all the equipment is working properly. This is not what concerns me at the moment; I am referring to the test of the actual procedures to be used in the experiment, interviewing, assessment, recording of data, etc.

During the preliminary trial, the data should be collected in exactly the same way as in the planned experiment and it is extremely valuable experience to run a statistical test on the data obtained. In this way one has an opportunity of seeing whether the material is amenable to analysis, what it means, and one has an opportunity of learning the particular techniques of statistical analysis. Furthermore, the data can be used to estimate the number of subjects that will be required, as I will show later. Those who are inexperienced in clinical research have a tendency to collect too much data; and when I say too much, I mean too much, i.e. more than they need. The net result is that, in the first place, they find it impossible to deal with the data that has been accumulated, and secondly, some of it may be of such nature that it cannot be analysed. The preliminary run, therefore, enables them to get rid of a good deal of this superfluous material.

During the preliminary trial one should remember that although one is at the stage of experimentation, one should still continue the process of observation. This should be done all the time, not only because it is useful practice but because now for the first time one begins to get a real understanding of the literature. When you are involved in the work yourself, when you are observing what is going on and seeing the difficulties, then much of what you have read begins to have a much clearer meaning. I have experienced this myself on many occasions.

The preliminary run may also show that your hypothesis is inadequate and may need to be revised. Some of the first findings may even suggest big changes in the experimental design, as well as in the hypothesis. Nevertheless, there are limits to this. A point is reached when you must make up your mind about what you are going to do and how you are going to do it. It is quite certain that whatever you do will suffer from defects, for perfection is impossible to achieve. In any case, there are always different ways of tackling the problem you are studying, taking into account different factors or different alternatives. You must use your judgement here and decide what you will take into acount, and what you will ignore and leave to another experiment. Once again, this is a matter for the clinician, and only another clinician can help him. If in doubt, always go to someone with appropriate experience for help and advice. You don't have to accept the advice (after all, your advisor may not know all the circumstances) but if you reject it, you will know why you have done so, and will then be in a better position to justify your investigation in the face of criticism.

Randomization

A clinical experiment is designed to compare two or more treatments. To ensure an unbiased comparison, it is necessary to allocate the subjects to the different treatments by some method of ' randomization '. This forms the basis, in the experiment, for the proper application of the theory of probability. At some suitable place in the experiment, subjects must be allocated to the treatments by chance. Where this occurs depends upon the design of the experiment. If it is a simple comparison between two or more groups, each of which is given a different treatment, then the subjects are allocated randomly to the groups. If it is a more complex design then the rule is that the randomization occurs within each unit experiment. For example, if three treatments are going to be compared on two different types of subjects, then the randomization is made separately for each type of subject.

Some investigators experience difficulties here. When the experiment is concerned with the evaluation of therapeutic procedures on sick patients then they begin to have doubts. They may have come to accept the need for proper control series but then they reject randomization because they feel it is wrong to do this. This is a mistaken belief, but it is important to be quite clear why it should be so. Given that some new therapy or therapeutic procedure appears likely to benefit patients, then it is a tradition of medicine, and a very old one, that it should be tried out. In the past, there has always been some enthusiast who has been willing to use the new treatment on a group of patients. The result of this was that the treatment was in fact tried out but in such a way that it could not be properly evaluated. For the patients it was a matter of chance if it was their physician who was the one who tried out the treatment or if they were included in the group on whom the treatment was tested. Randomization does not introduce chance, it does so in such a way that real information can be obtained. The long history of the introduction of new remedies which were eventually found to be useless or even harmful is, in the end, the justification for the setting up of a control series and proper allocation to different treatments.

Random allocation means that there is an equal chance for any one of the subjects to receive any one of the treatments to be tested. If it has to be done it should be done properly. To allocate alternative subjects, where there are two treatments, is not a satisfactory substitute for randomization. Experience has shown that once the investigator decides to use alternative allocation then there will be a conspiracy by all those working with him, or connected with the patients, assistants, nurses, secretaries, G.P.'s and others, to push particular patients into a favoured treatment and to ensure that they do not receive a treatment which is disapproved of. I have also seen investigators trying to 'invent' an imitation of a random allocation! I cannot understand why there should be so much resistance to doing a randomization properly but I have to accept the fact that it does exist.

The simplest and most obvious method for randomization into two groups is to toss a coin. If there are four groups, then the coin is tossed to determine whether the individual goes into groups 1 and 2 or groups 3 and 4, and then the coin is tossed again for the final decision. It is more difficult to toss a coin in order to randomize into an odd number of groups but it can be done. Nevertheless, tossing a coin, say 50 times, and recording the results takes a very long time and is surprisingly laborious. The best and most convenient way is to use a table of random numbers. Such a table is constructed carefully and then tested to ensure that in the long run all the numbers from 0 to 9 appear equally often and the occurrence of any one is independent of the previous one.

Pick out any row and column in the table and find the number where they intersect. Then move along the row or column and when you reach the end go on to the next one. If the number in the table is odd then you record group 1 and if it is even you record group 2; zero counts as even. The subjects in the list are then allocated in order as recorded. If there are three groups, you ignore the zero when you find it in the table and go on to the next number. Then if the number in the table is 1, 4 or 7 the subject goes into group 1, if it is 2, 5 or 8 into group 2, and if 3, 6 or 9 into group 3. The rule is to divide the number in the table by 3 and the remainder gives the group number. If there are four groups, you ignore the numbers zero and 1 in the table. Divide the number in the table by 4 and the remainder gives the group number. Thus 2 and 6 go into group 2, 3 and 7 go to group 3, 4 and 8 go to group 4, 5 and 9 go into group 1. An alternative way is to do the randomization in two stages. If the number is odd then the subject goes into the odd groups 1 and 3, and if the number is even the subject goes into the even groups 2 and 4. When you have randomized all the subjects you then go through them again, to decide to which of each pair of groups the subject is allocated. For five groups, use all the ten numbers 0 to 9. For six groups, use the method for three groups, and repeat each as for two groups. For seven groups, ignore 0, 8 and 9. For eight groups, use the method for four groups and repeat for two. For nine groups ignore the zero and then the numbers give the group number. I think it is unlikely that you will ever want to use ten or more groups but if you should do so you will have to work out the method for yourself!

An experiment is always most efficient if there are equal numbers of subjects in each of the groups, hence allocation is random but with a restriction. This is done by going through the table until one group is completed. All the other subjects are then randomized to the other groups. When all but one of the groups are completed the rest of the subjects go into the last group.

This method is most suitable when all the subjects are available at the same time, e.g. all the patients in a ward. When all the subjects are not immediately available and you have to wait for them to appear, e.g. a particular type of patient, it will be more convenient to divide the total number of subjects into ' blocks ' and to be sure that the numbers in the different groups are equal within the blocks. It may be that you have decided to use 50 subjects in your experiment and then for some reason or other it is necessary to stop before you have reached the total. If you have ensured that there are equal numbers of subjects for the treatment in blocks of, say, 8 or 10, then no harm is done if you have to stop the experiment at, say, 40 cases.

Controls

A question that causes much debate is one concerning the control series. In a trial of a new drug, should the control series receive a placebo or another drug? Obviously, this depends on the question that is being asked in the trial, i.e. does the treatment have any effect at all, or is it better than standard treatment? I would say that, for practical purposes, the control series should receive the accepted standard treatment for their disorder. Medicine has been practised for a long time (contrary to popular belief, it is the oldest profession) and what we want to know usually is whether the new is better than the old. There is one advantage in giving the control series a placebo, and that is, in this way it is easier to determine the *ill effects* of the treatments. There is one circumstance in which a placebo control must be used, and that is when we are using an untried method of assessment. It is always possible that a null result may signify, not that the treatments do not differ significantly in their effects, but that method of assessment is insensitive to the differences. If, however, one of the active treatments is significantly different from the placebo controls, using the particular method of assessment, then this settles the matter.

Another problem concerns the subject of ' natural ' controls. When we wish to investigate the effects of a ' natural ' experiment, e.g. the effects of diet, occupation, habitat, exercise or mode of life, on some disorder or other problem we are interested in, we obtain our control series by trying to find subjects who are like those under observation in every respect except the one under consideration. Of course, we can consider two or more factors using a factorial design.

Such a situation is fraught with difficulties. In the type of investigation I have been concerned with, we *make* our control series, and if we have done the job properly, we know that our groups are truly comparable in the sense that they permit an unbiased comparison. When we have to find our control series, we cannot be certain that our two groups *are* comparable. This does not mean that we have to give up the attempt, for it may be the only way that is available to us of obtaining the information we want. A very important example of such an investigation was the inquiry that showed that cigarette smoking was associated with the development of cancer of the lungs. When a control series has to be found, it is very important that the investigator should endeavour to demonstrate that the controls are like the observed series, in as many factors as are thought to be relevant.

Of course, one cannot demonstrate that the control series is *like* the experimental series, what one does is to do a statistical test which determines whether the two groups could be regarded as being random samples from the same population. It is also very useful to do this in every experiment which entails a random allocation to different treatments, to see what effect the randomization has had, before going on to analyse the results of the experiment. One should examine the differences between the groups on those variables which could be considered to have an influence on the results. It could be argued that such variables should have been taken into account in the design but there are limits to what can be done in one experiment. In practice, you consider the important variables and either eliminate them by selection, or include them as factors, the rest you abandon to be included as part of normal variation. Sooner or later, the process of randomization will produce unexpected differences between groups and this becomes all the more certain the more variables one examines. If statistically significant differences are found, this does not mean that the experiment is wrong or should be abandoned. If the experiment was properly designed and the randomization properly carried out, then the experiment is a good one and its results stand. If some of the groups show significant differences, then this means that inferences about the results of the experiment should be made with caution.

The 'Blind' Trial

This is a suitable moment to deal with the 'blind' trial. I have the impression sometimes that the belief in the 'blind' trial is becoming a superstition. The 'blind' trial must not be confused with the 'controlled' trial. As I have pointed out to you before, a trial of treatment is always a comparison of differences, the differences between two or more treatments. One of the 'treatments' may be nothing at all, but this is uncommon. Even interviewing and investigating a patient may have a profound effect on his morale and this will show itself in his symptoms and his reactions to them. Admitting a patient to hospital, even if only for investigations, will have a greater effect, and so will rest in bed. Such a comparison is fundamental, and the purpose of the controlled trial is to ensure that the comparison is made in such a way that valid conclusions can be drawn.

If I want to compare the effectiveness of two haematinics, I can do so by taking a group of patients suffering from anaemia, and allotting them randomly to the two treatments. Better still, I could match them in pairs according to the severity of the anaemia, and randomly allot one of each pair to a treatment and the other of the pair to the other treatment. I arrange for the patients to receive their treatments, and then at some suitable interval or intervals I take a sample of blood and measure the concentration of haemoglobin on the usual photoelectric haemoglobinometer. This is a controlled trial, but not a 'blind' trial. If, in a trial, I use as criterion of improvement the patient's symptoms or some subjective change within him, it is necessary that the patients should not know which treatment they are receiving, as this may bias their answers when questioned about their condition. That is the 'single blind' trial, and it is quite adequate if the method of questioning is standardized and objective, e.g. by questionnaire. If the assessment of the patients' condition has to be done by the physician, then the results he will obtain may be determined by his attitude, e.g. his belief or disbelief in the new treatment. In such a case it is important that the physician should not know which patient has received treatment. This is the 'double blind' trial. The term is used generally to imply that all the patients' attendants are 'blind' in this way. There have been attempts to introduce the term 'triple blind', but this is quite unnecessary. My own opinion is that this term should be reserved for those trials where the investigators do not know what they are doing or why!

It has been said sometimes that a double blind trial is not really blind, because the presence of the active treatment can be detected by its side effects. To overcome this, it has been suggested that the control series should be given some drug which will produce similar side-effects. The ethics of this are doubtful and it also gives rise to another difficulty. I can remember a controlled trial where a traditional treatment was tested against a very careful imitation. The result showed that the accepted treatment was not significantly different from the imitation. Some critics of this investigation suggested that the result could be interpreted as proving that the imitation was also an effective treatment! Perhaps it would have been better to have included a group which did not receive any form of treatment.

In order to ensure that a controlled trial is truly blind, it is important to make the different treatments resemble each other as closely as possible and it is necessary to ensure that the actual treatment given to a patient is kept secret. Usually it is not difficult to make the treatments resemble each other but sometimes considerable ingenuity may be required to do so. I was once asked how it would be possible to compare an inhalation anaesthetic with an injectable one, in a blind trial, and I replied that this could be done by giving every patient a gas to inhale and also an injection. In one group the gas would be an anesthetic and the injection would be a dummy or an injection of saline, and in the other case the injection would be the anaesthetic and the gas would be air or oxygen. I also pointed out that this raised a difficulty concerning the ethics of giving unnecessary injections. When it comes to different surgical operations or different interviewing techniques or types of treatment which are radically different in their nature, then it is obviously impossible to make them look alike. Certainly, for those who are carrying out the treatment it is impossible not to know which one has been given. In such cases, it is sufficient to ensure that the assessment of the results of the treatment is carried out in ignorance of the nature of the treatment. In other words, whoever does the assessment does not carry out the treatment and vice versa.

The simplest procedure for maintaining ' blindness ' is that found in a drug trial where all the patients are immediately available. The patients are first given case numbers and a list is made of these numbers. These are then randomly allocated to the different groups as I have already dscribed. The list is then handed to the pharmacist who allots the group to treatments by some method of randomization. He dispenses the drugs by putting them into bottles labelled with the name of the patient. The most complicated procedure applies to a factorial design comparing different treatments, when the subjects are not immediately available and the nature of the treatments is obvious. Case numbers are first randomly distributed to the rows and then the cases in each row are randomly distributed to the columns. With factors which are not experimental but are concerned with the attributes of the subject, e.g. sex or social status, it is convenient to give a separate series of case numbers for each category. For example, the male cases would run from 0 to 99 and the females from 100 to 199. The next step is better done by somebody who is not concerned with the selection of subjects. The rows and columns of the design are then randomly allocated to the treatments. Finally, take a note-pad or book and on each sheet write a case number. On the back of the sheet write the treatment for that case number. The sheets are then stapled together so that it is not possible to determine which treatment a particular case number will receive until the sheet is torn out of the note book. The treatment is described by a code letter and the pharmacist dispenses the appropriate treatment. Each treatment should have several code letters.

It is very important to discuss with all those concerned the full details of the procedure and make sure that everybody understands it and is willing to follow the procedure correctly. At the same time it is very useful to try to find out in what way the procedure could be disorganized. It is surprising how easy it is for things to go wrong and a little thought beforehand will save much anxiety afterwards.

I have already pointed out that the first stage of an investigation should, if possible, be considered as a trial run. If this can be done, you must arrange the allocation of patients in such a way that it is possible to determine the treatments given to the subjects in the trial run with breaking the 'blindness' for the rest of the subjects.

Ethics of Therapeutic Trials

Since I have mentioned the subject of medical ethics, I ought to say something about the ethics of controlled trials. It is often argued that it is unethical for a physician to deprive some of his patients of the benefits of the new treatment, in order to produce a control series. I think that the argument is standing on its head. The real problem is not whether the physician should refrain from giving some of his patients a new and untried drug, but whether he is ethically justified in *giving* it to some of his patients. Again and again, as soon as a new treatment is introduced, within a short period I have seen reports of its effect, it having been administered to scores and even hundreds of patients. These reports are not controlled and they are generally very enthusiastic over their remarkable results! If only these investigators had refrained from exposing half their patients to the alleged benefits (and dangers) or the new treatment, we would have solid informaion abou its value. When the new treatments are drugs, I have often heard complaints about this made against the manufacturers, but the fault lies with the medical profession as a whole, and the editors of medical journals in particular. It would be a great help if they insisted on high standards, and refused to publish anything which fell below these standards, however eminent the authors might be.

The ethics of therapeutic trials is far too big a subject for me to consider in adequate detail, so I shall confine myself to some of the fundamental principles. The first rule is that the patients' interests must be safeguarded. We must remember that, however much care we take over the planning, a therapeutic trial can not mean the same to the patients as the routine administration of a standard treatment. We must expect that patients will be exposed to some risk however slight, they may undergo some trouble and even expense, and the trial may involve them having to wait longer than absolutely necessary for their treatment. We must recognize our responsibilities and do the utmost we can not to break faith with those who trust us. A therapeutic trial can always be carried out without interfering with the rights of patients, and if this does not seem possible then it has been badly designed. I suppose that there must be some cases where it cannot be redesigned and in that case the trial should be abandoned. Ask yourself if you would object, if you found yourself or a near relative included in the trial. Would you be prepared to defend your behaviour in public? If you are in any doubt, consult your colleagues. Most hospitals now have a special ' Ethical Committee ' which will pass an opinion on any project. The committee's judgement should be an adequate safeguard, but the ultimate responsibility is that of the investigator.

One of the most important aspects of the planning of a clinical investigation and especially a therapeutic trial, is the setting up of a ' fail-safe ' procedure. Try to think of anything that could conceivably go wrong in such way as to cause inconvenience to your subjects or even worse, and then try to devise some way of dealing with it. The first 'fail safe' procedure in a double-blind trial is to arrange that it should be possible to find out what treatment a particular subject is receiving. You must make sure that the information can be obtained without delay by anybody who is concerned, and you should make sure that everybody knows how to obtain it quickly. While you are about it, you should make sure that although the 'key' can be broken for a particular individual it is not thereby broken for everybody.

If a patient develops unwanted side-effects from a drug, the dose should be cut immediately. This is why it is so much better to use a flexible system of dosage and to co-operate with a colleague who will adjust doses appropriately. The patient can thereby receive an appropriate dose and not be lost to the trial. It is always useful to make arrangements which will prevent the loss of data from patients who have to leave the trial. You could assess them when they leave or give an arbitrary assessment of 'no improvement' or 'condition unchanged'. This should be explained in the report of the trial and, if there are only a few such cases, no harm will have been done; if there are many, the trial was badly planned.

Summary

This lecture has been concerned with certain practical aspects of a clinical investigation. The first part should be so planned that it can act as a 'trial run' and permit of alterations. The details of randomization and the principles and practice of double-blind trials were described. The ethics of therapeutic trials have been considered and the opinion given that proper planning can ensure that there is no contravention of ethical principles.

The Criterion

In previous lectures, I have on various occasions made references to the criterion of change. In this lecture, I intend to bring together this matter and consider further important and practical aspects. In clinical research, the purpose of an experiment is to produce a change in a subject by means of a treatment. In most cases, we can measure the state of the subject before and after the treatment; in 'natural experiments' we usually can measure only the state after the 'treatment'. Since any treatment to a biological system will produce many changes, it is necessary first to decide which ones will be measured. The choice will obviously depend on the relevance of a particular criterion to the investigator's interests.

Relevance of Criterion

A clinician is not often concerned with the problem of the appropriateness of his criterion. Patients come to him because they are suffering from symptoms, and his aim is to diminish or eliminate them, preferably by eliminating the causative disease. It must be remembered that a treatment could diminish a patient's symptoms without necessarily improving his capacity to cope with the problems of life, e.g. earning a living, or even merely staying out of hospital. In the treatment of chronic schizophrenia, it is really more important to get the patient into a condition where he can leave hospital and go out and earn his living and live with his family, than it is to diminish his hallucinations or delusions. After all, there are many people outside mental hospitals who are suffering from delusions and hallucinations. Nobody would want to keep them in a mental hospital just for that.

An example from general medicine will illustrate what I mean about the problems of the relevance of criterion. When anticoagulant drugs were first introduced as a 'treatment' for coronary thrombosis, they roused tremendous interest. A great spate of research followed, in which many drugs were tested and much ingenuity was exerted to devise methods of measuring their effect. Nevertheless, I often wondered if all that effort had been somewhat displaced. It seemed to me that the real criterion was not the maintenance of a low coagulability of the blood, but the incidence of recurrence of thrombosis and, ultimately, the death rate or expectation of life. In due course, researches were published which had used these criteria and, unfortunately, the results were shown to be much less good than had been hoped for. Enthusiasm for this form of treatment has now diminished considerably. I am not just decrying laboratory tests, but I am trying to bring out the relevance of clinical criteria to clinical problems. The fact that I am a psychiatrist gives me a bias in favour of over-all clinical results rather than laboratory tests, but I have yet to be convinced that the general well-being of a patient is not the most fundamental and the most practical of criteria by which to judge a treatment.

The psychiatrist has no other criteria, because mental diseases are disturbances of the whole person, they interfere with his social relationships and activities (of course, they also interfere with his subjective well-being). Any derangements of the patient's physiology are incidental in most mental disorders, whereas they are the essence of general medical and surgical diseases. It is for this reason that interest is concentrated on laboratory tests as a criterion of the effectiveness of treatment. There is another reason often given, which is mistaken, but I shall deal with it later.

Measurements of the criterion may be direct or indirect. Examples of the latter are the measurement of oxygen saturation of the blood in the ear instead of in the brain, arm-to-arm circulation time, and so on. Direct measurements are usually obvious, but the distinction between the two types is not always clear. Which is the more and which the less direct criterion for treatment of angina: changes in the ECG or in exercise tolerance? It is important to remember that the use of instruments may convert a direct measurement into an indirect one. Indirect measurements always suffer from the introduction of additional sources of error, but provided such error can be kept small, they may be better than direct measurements for all sorts of reasons. In my own field of work, direct measurements are always subjective judgements. Attempts have been made to introduce the use of psychological tests, but although such indirect measurements are of great value, because they can be scored objectively, their relevance is always to some extent in doubt.

A problem closely related to the relevance of measurements is the frequency with which they are made. I am often asked how frequently measurements of improvement should be made and my answer is: as infrequently as possible, taking into account the information that is required. To measure the improvement due to treatment, all one needs is a 'before' and 'after' measurement. If such measurements are insufficiently reliable, i.e. they have too much error, then both the 'before' and 'after' measurements should be repeated two or more times (and the average taken) to reduce the error below the desired level. If you want to find out when improvement takes place, then you should make your measurements before and after the time when you think it takes place. The exact times depend on how much prior information you have, and how accurately you want to know the time of change. If you are interested in the rate of change, then two measurements at suitable intervals will give you the necessary information, provided that you can assume that the rate is constant, i.e. that the change can be represented by a straight line. If this is unlikely, you will need more measurements to determine the changes in the rate. If you can assume that the changes can be represented by some mathematical curve and you want to determine its nature, then the number of measurements required will depend on the parameters of the curve, e.g. a parabola requires at least three measurements.

Objective and Subjective Assessments

In clinical medicine, it is often said that when one can choose among different methods of measuring the effect of treatment one should always use an objective measure. The reasons given for this choice are usually that objective measures are unaffected by observer's bias and that in any case they are somehow more 'real'. The choice is correct but the reasons are wrong. There is much misunderstanding of the problem. Many 'objective' measures are really subjective. The usual method of measuring blood pressure depends upon the judgement of the observer of the moment of appearance of certain sounds in the stethoscope, or their disappearance or change in quality. When we measure the strength of grip, the range of movement at a joint or the vital capacity of a patient, we are depending upon the subjective state of the patient; the result obtained will depend on his mood and interest. Of course the expectations of the observer and of the subject will introduce bias but there are plenty of ways of diminishing this. When one is measuring some underlying disturbance of body chemistry, then the appropriate techniques have to be used and these are usually objective. In other situations, the reason for using instrumental methods of measurement is that they reduce the errors of measurement.

Errors of measurement constitute a source of variation additional to all others, and much of the point of the design of experiments is to diminish such natural variation. The accuracy of instruments may be spurious and misleading. No matter how accurately an instrument may measure the amount of haemoglobin in the blood, if the method of obtaining the blood does not yield a representative sample, and if the syringes which measure the quantity of the sample are themselves not accurate, then the result will be false. When we measure the daily excretion of steroids in the urine, the accuracy of our instruments may be completely nullified if we cannot be sure that the sample tested really is the full 24-hour excretion of the kidneys.

When we want to measure disturbances of function, we will often find that objective measures are usually nothing more than indices and even then not very good ones. When we study Parkinsonism, we can easily and objectively measure the amount of tremor and rigidity in muscles, but how much do these reflect the disability suffered by the patient? What matters about a measurement is the amount of information it gives us. A pulse rate can be measured as objectively and as accurately as we wish but it does not tell us much about the function of the heart.

Reliability and Validity

What matters about a measurement is not whether it is objective or subjective, but whether it gives us the information we require. This can be considered on two aspects: a given technique should give measurements which reflect the changes in the function in which we are interested or, as it is sometimes put, a measure should measure what it is supposed to measure! The results of our observations should also be trustworthy. In technical terms, a measurement should have high validity and reliability.

The problems of validity and reliability are extremely complicated and it would not be appropriate for me to go into them in detail. I already touched on them when I considered the relevance of the criterion. As far as you are concerned, you can ignore the question of validity if you use an accepted measure for your criterion. It is when you use a new method, or a new variation of an accepted method, of measuring the criterion that it will be necessary for you to establish its validity. In general, you will use two methods: group differentiation and the effects of experimental factors. In the first case you will take two or more groups who out to differ with respect to the criterion you are measuring and then demonstrate with your measurements that they do indeed differ. In the second, you have to demonstrate that the effects of a treatment show changes in your criterion of the sort that you would expect. For example, if you wish to measure the relative effectiveness of two treatments, then by introducing a third group which is not given any treatment you can demonstrate whether your criterion is valid. There may or may not be significant differences between the results of the two treatments, but if at least one treatment is significantly different from no treatment then clearly your criterion of measurement is a valid one. As for reliability, the simplest way to establish that is to repeat your measurements. If you obtain the same results on both occasions, or very similar ones, then your measures have good reliability. Both validity and reliability can be measured quantitatively in terms of correlations, which I shall describe in due course.

Types of Criterion

For convenience, I have classified the criterion into four types, though I have no doubt there are many other and better ways.

The first type is one in which a ' final ' state appears, which was not present beforehand. Examples of such are sea-sickness, where the aim of the treatment is to prevent the appearance of the symptoms. The same applies to post-anaesthetic vomiting. Another type would be the trial of treatment to shorten parturition. This is particularly so in primiparae, where we have no previous experience to go on. I have already dealt with this type of experiment. The procedure is to allot patients randomly to the two groups and measure the amount of presence of the state which is the criterion, e.g. the presence or severity of vomiting, or the length of labour.

The second type of criterion is that in which the ' final state ' is always achieved. An example of such is the use of a haematinic for the treatment of anaemia. I do not know of any such which will not eventually bring the concentration of haemoglobin up to normal. In this case, we could use the rate of improvement as our criterion. The use of anticoagulants for the prevention of recurrence of coronary thrombosis is another such example. Since we can reduce the coagulability of the blood to any level we wish, by giving an appropriate dose, the criterion might be the steadiness with which we could maintain the level required. We could then give the different drugs in the doses required to produce the given level, and measure this at regular intervals. The mean level for the different drugs would be the same, but we would measure the variability, and test for the difference between variances. Much the same might be done when comparing different insulins, using the variability of blood-sugar. For a condition like duodenal ulcer, where adequate treatment and rest will usually end with the healing of the ulcer, we could use the time required for healing as our criterion, or the time until relapse.

In those cases were the ' final state ' is not always achieved, e.g. in a trial of antibiotics, we could obviously use the proportion of recoveries as criterion, and our statistical test would be on the differences between proportions.

The fourth type is one in which the ' final state ' differs quantitatively from the initial state of the subject. Thus in rheumatoid arthritis we would not expect all disability to disappear; in chronic schizophrenia we do not usually obtain more than a partial amelioration of symptoms. We therefore have, at the end of our experiment, two scores for each subject, one before and one after treatment. What is the best way of using our data?

Properties of Criterion

You will not be surprised if I say that it all depends on what you want to know. For convenience of exposition, I shall assume that your data is derived from a therapeutic trial. The criterion is some sort of measurement of severity of symptoms, so complete recovery gives a zero score. There are four ways in which you can handle the pair of numbers obtained for each patient. (1) Final score. You ignore the initial score and the statistical analysis deals only with the final scores. (2) Difference scores. Subtract the final score from the initial score (since the former is usually less than the latter) and use the difference score for your statistical analysis. (3) Ratio score. The final score is expressed as a percentage of the initial score. (4) Analysis of covariance. This is a statistical technique, which I shall explain in due course, which takes into account the initial score of each subject and eliminates its influence on the final score.

The final score is a direct measurement and is a clear index of a patient's condition. It enables you to compare one patient with another and to compare one group with another. This is not true of the other kinds of scores. If you are interested in the amount of improvement, then the difference score gives you this information. It is important to recognize that there are two limitations to the information given by a difference score. In the first place, a patient who is only mildly ill and starts off with a low score can obtain only a small amount of improvement as shown by a difference score, whereas a more severely ill patient can show a greater improvement. This contradicts the basic assumption that the effect of the treatment is the same for all individuals in the group. This is not such a serious problem as may first appear as it applies equally to all the treatments being compared, but it does mean that one must be wary of comparing difference scores between one patient and another. If, however, you use a ratio score, the amount of improvement possible to patients is made the same for all of them. Difference scores that are equal are not necessarily equivalent. Thus a drop from 50 points to 40 points is not necessarily the same, in clinical significance, as a drop of 15 to 5 points. This is true even if the scores represent objective physical measurements. If you want to distinguish clearly between those patients who have made a complete recovery and those who have not, you must use either the final or ratio scores. If you want to identify clearly those patients whose condition is unchanged or even worse, you must use difference or ratio scores. A ratio score is therefore the best index to use when you want to measure responsiveness to treatment.

The variability of the initial state of patients may be a factor which influences the final state. It can therefore interfere with and obscure the effects of the treatments. One way of eliminating this is to select the patients so that they are all of approximately the same amount of severity. A better way, as I have pointed out, is to classify them into separate levels of severity and to use these levels as a factor in a factorial design. Another method is to use the statistical technique of analysis of covariance which takes into account the initial state of the subjects and eliminates it from the final result. This avoids the arbitrary division into grades of severity but is itself subject to certain limitations. I shall return to the subject in a subsequent lecture and consider it in relation to an actual example.

This is a very brief and inadequate account of the four methods of dealing with the criterion score. If you should ever need to consider them in relation to a practical problem, you can look up the reference (given after the summary) for more information.

Distribution of Criterion

The statistical analysis of data is concerned with the means of groups, and the final test of significance determines the probability of the null hypothesis, based on the assumption that the distribution of means is a Gaussian or related distribution. You have already seen that the distribution of means is close to a Gaussian distribution, even if the distribution of the original data is not. Nevertheless, it is always useful to know that the original data do have a distribution bearing some resemblance to a Gaussian one, i.e. high in the middle and low at the two ends. As long as the distribution of your data is reasonably symmetrical, the estimation of probabilities is reasonably good, but difficulties arise when the central hump is not in the middle. The commonest deviation from this, found in biology, is where the central hump is far to the left, i.e. high values occur with excessive frequency, as illustrated in Figure 11.1.

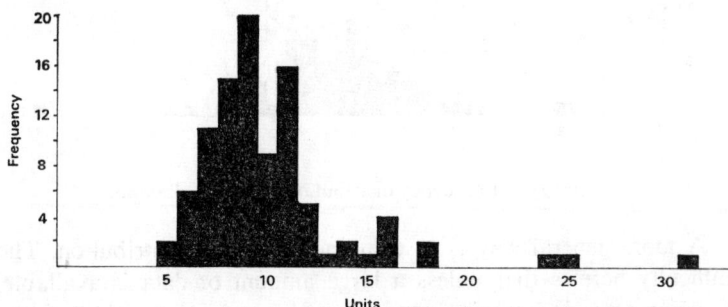

Figure 11.1. Frequency distribution of alkaline phosphatase in blood (97 cases).

The simplest way to 'normalize' such a distribution is to transform the data by taking the logarithms of the original scores. This changes equal proportionate increases into equal increments. For example, the numbers 10, 100, 1,000 and 10,000 show equal proportionate increases. When converted into logarithms to the base 10, they become 1, 2, 3, and 4, which show equal increments. Such a transformation is not uncommon; dosages of drugs and blood concentration are usually thought of in these terms, e.g. increasing from 5 to 10 mg is regarded as equivalent to increasing from 20 to 40 or from 100 to 200 mg. To give an actual example, doses of 1, 2, 5 and 10 mg of trifluoperazine are regarded as equivalent more or less to doses of chlorpromazine ranging through 25, 50, 125, and 250 mg.

It will be always worthwhile to examine your data and look at the distribution. A short cut method is to examine the data in the different groups, e.g. cells in a two-way design. Calculate the means and the variances, or standard deviations, of each group, then place the means in ascending order and their variances with them. Compare the way in which the variances change. If the variances are also in ascending order (more or less) then a logarithmic transformation is probably required.

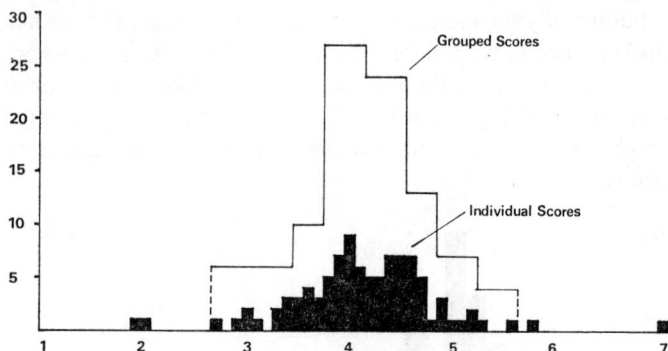

Figure 11.2. Frequency distribution of serum albumin.

A more general way is to examine the actual distribution. The difficulty here is that unless a large amount of data is available, the histogram is irregular anyway, as shown in Figure 11.2. Some of the irregularity can be smoothed out by grouping together all the cases within a given range of scores, as shown in the figure, but the result is still unsatisfactory usually. An even better way is to plot the cumulative distribution as in Figure 11.3. This has one great advantage, that there is no need to group together the scores and each score can be taken separately. A cumulative distribution gives an S-shaped curve but it is still difficult to tell whether it is reasonably close to a Gaussian distribution. The best method of all is to plot the cumulative distribution on probability graph paper which converts the Gaussian distribution into a straight line. One slight difficulty is that neither 0 per cent nor 100 per cent can be plotted on such graph paper as the former in an infinite distance to the left and the latter an infinite distance to the right. A slight adjustment of the cumulative distribution is therefore necessary.

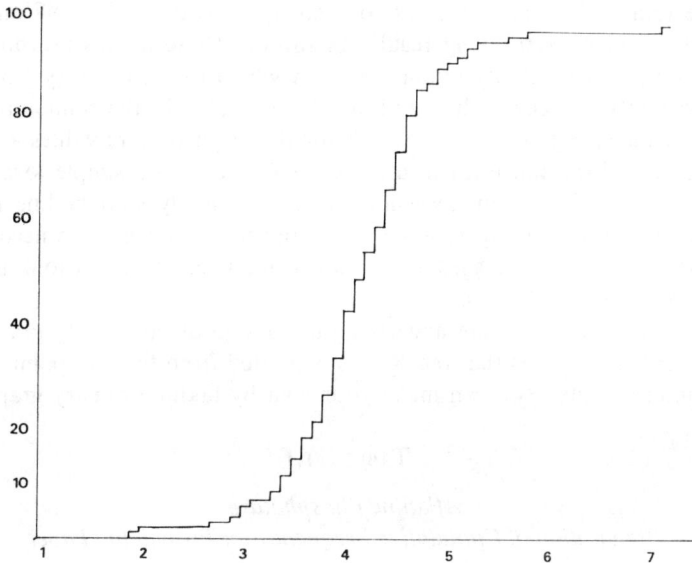

Figure 11.3. Cumulative frequency distribution of serum albumin.

This is done by preparing a table containing five columns and filling in the first three from the data, as in Table 11.1. The first column contains the actual scores, the second contains their frequency and the third the cumulative frequency. The next step requires making the assumption that a given score represents really a range of scores, and that all the subjects with that score are evenly distributed along that range. Thus scores of 1, 2, 3, etc., are equivalent to 0·5 to 1·4, 1·5 to 2·4, 2·5 to 3·4, etc. Theoretically, there are also scores of 0·4 downwards and 3·5 upwards, but as there are no cases in them they are therefore ignored when plotting the distribution. To complete the fourth column in the table of ' adjusted cumulative frequency ' the procedure is as follows : all the cases with score of 5 units are assumed to be evenly spaced between 4·5 and 5·4. The total number of cases up to a score of 5 units is therefore all the scores below, i.e. zero, plus half of the cases lying between 4·5 and 5·4. 0+2/2=1. The total number of cases up to score 6 units is all those below plus half in the range 5·5 to 6·4. This is 2+6/2=5. This is repeated for each value of the score and column 4 is completed in this way. It will be seen that half of the cases in the last score (value 31 units) are lost. The last column is filled in by converting these adjusted cumulative frequencies into percentages of the total. There are 97 cases so each figure is divided by 97 and multiplied by 100 giving results as shown. These figures are now plotted on probability graph paper, in which the ordinate (y axis) represents the score values and the abscissa (X axis) the cumulative percentage. Figure 11.4 shows this for the original score values and for the values transformed into their logarithms. If a simple logarithmic transformation does not give a reasonably straight line in probability graph paper, some other transformation may be necessary. If so I would suggest that you consult a statistician or look up a text book on statistics.

What is the principle underlying the design of probability graph paper? the basis is that the X axis is plotted from the mid-point in standard units. You can make your own by taking ordinary graph

TABLE 11.1

Alkaline Phosphatase
Preparation of Cumulative Frequency for Probability Paper

Score	Frequency	Cumulative frequency	Adjusted Cumulative frequency	Adjus. Cum. frequency %
5	2	2	1	1·0
6	6	8	5	5·2
7	11	19	13·5	13·9
8	15	34	26·5	27·3
9	20	54	44	45·4
10	9	63	58·5	60·3
11	16	79	71	73·2
12	5	84	81·5	84·0
13	1	85	84·5	87·1
14	2	87	86	88·7
15	1	88	87·5	90·2
16	4	92	90	92·8
18	2	94	93	95·9
24	1	95	94·5	97·4
25	1	96	95·5	98·4
31	1	97	96·5	99·5

paper, marking the mid point of the X axis as zero and then marking to the left and right in standard deviation units. Mark the points in tenths of a unit running from -2.5 to $+2.5$ (this should be sufficient for most purposes). Then, from the table of the normal (Gaussian) distribution, convert these into cumulative percentages. Thus zero is equivalent to 50 per cent, 1.0 is equivalent to $50+34.1$ $=84.1$ per cent, -1.0 is equivalent to $50-34.1=15.9$ per cent, and so on. The percentages thus marked are rather awkward figures and probability graph paper marks more convenient ones, e.g. 5 per cent, 10 per cent, 20 per cent, 30 per cent etc. You can do it yourself if you are prepared to go to the trouble.

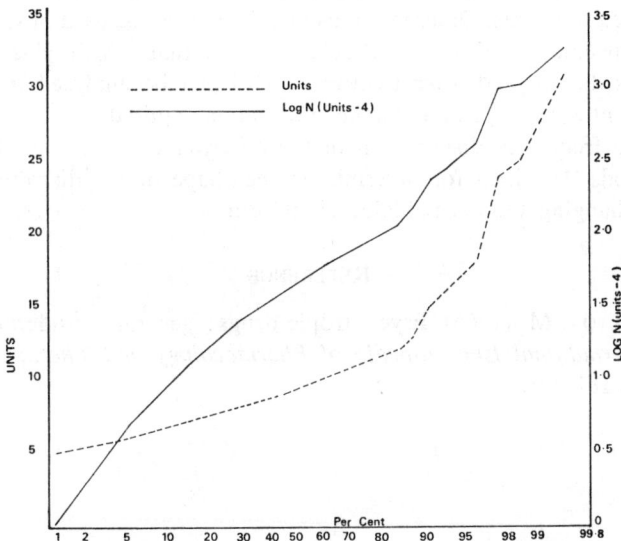

Figure 11.4. Cumulative frequency of alkaline phosphatase.

What makes this technique so useful is that it will work even if the number of cases is relatively small, if the scores are irregularly spaced and finally, if there is only one case for each score value. The scores should be adjusted for differences between the group means and this is particularly important if the data comes from a factorial design, when they should be adjusted for differences between the cell means. In each cell, the difference between the cell mean and the general mean is calculated and this is algebraically added (i.e. subtracted if negative) to the scores in the cells. No great accuracy is needed. It is sufficient if the adjustment is made so that cell means are now within one unit of each other.

Summary

The chief advantage of objective over subjective criteria is that by using suitable instruments the errors of measurement can be decreased without limit, but this may not be important if other sources of error are greater. Subjective assessments are liable to much error and bias but these can be decreased as required.

A criterion of change should be relevant to the purpose required and should have high validity and reliability. These are the important requirements. Different kinds of criterion can be used in various circumstances and one particular type is that which gives two scores, before and after treatment. This can be analysed in four different ways, depending on the information required.

The frequency distribution of the criterion was considered and methods described for determining the shape of the distributions and changing it to normal (Gaussian) form.

REFERENCE

HAMILTON, M. (1966). Psychotropic drugs: general considerations. *International Encyclopedia of Pharmacology and Therapeutics*, **6,1,** 181-201.

Ranking and Rating Methods

One of the most important aspects of a clinical training is that it teaches the student not only what signs and symptoms to look for but how to perceive them. The clinician has to learn how to detect the signs of illness even in their mildest form. Admittedly, we use physical and biochemical tests to supplement our senses, but human perception is extraordinarily delicate and subtle and it is very easy to underestimate it. The ordinary man has no difficulty in distinguishing between a painting by Van Gogh and one by Rembrandt, but an art expert can take a brief look at a Rembrandt and tell in what year it was painted. A good clinician makes ample use of his perceptive powers and a good research worker should not neglect this source of information.

Ranking Methods

When the effects of a treatment produce a change in complex patterns of behaviour, symptoms or signs, then there are two ways in which such change can be assessed. We can disentangle the complex pattern into a number of single variables, assess them and then recombine them. Alternatively, we can use our judgement to assess the change as an entity. There is no difficulty in this and the practising clinician is doing it all the time in the course of his work, e.g. in deciding that one patient is more ill than another, or that the patient has improved or become worse. Faced with a group of patients he can place them in a rank order of increasing severity.

The method of ranking is an extremely simple and useful one for assessing the results of a clinical investigation. It is most useful when the criterion is present before and after treatment. A group of subjects is taken and put into rank order on the criterion. Since ranking, like any other form of measurement, is liable to error, you can reduce the error by repeating the ranking after a suitable interval (to diminish the effect of remembering the previous ranking). It takes much less time and gives better results if you can enlist the co-operation of one or more colleagues. Each of them does the ranking independently. You then calculate the means of these ranks for each subject and place the subjects in order of their mean ranking scores. This determines the final rank order of your subjects. Incidentally, it is simpler to use the totals rather than the means, since all the subjects will have the same number of rankings.

There are two alternative procedures at this point. In the first, the subjects can be randomly allocated to the treatments. The treatments are given and at the end of the experiment the ranking process is repeated. The changes in rank order can then be compared for the two treatments using an appropriate method of statistical analysis. The second method is to use the method of matched pairs. The subjects with ranks 1 and 2 form the first pair, the subjects with ranks 3 and 4 form the second pair and so on. By some method of randomization, one treatment is allotted to one member of the pair and the other to the other. At the end of the experiment, you then decide which one of each pair has shown the most change on the criterion. For the first treatment, this counts as a better or worse. Those pairs which show no difference in the effects of the treatments are ignored in the statistical analysis. The results are then analysed by the Sign test, the basis of which was described in Lecture 8. Let me give you an example using a complex indirect measure. Suppose we want to compare two treatments for Parkinsonism. We could do this by using the handwriting of the patients as criterion. We ask each patient to copy a short passage, and then these are ranked, say, according to legibility. On this basis, the patients are allotted to the treatments in the way I have just described, and at the end of the trial, they write the passage out again. These are then ranked and the changes analysed. If we are considering defects of speech and their improvement, we could record the reading of a given passage on tape, and use the same procedure with the tape recordings.

The great disadvantage of ranking methods is that it is difficult to rank many subjects. One solution to this difficulty is to rank the subjects in batches of, say, ten or twelve at a time. If the matched-pairs design is used, then all the data can be assembled into one group for analysis by the Sign test. Another way of coping with many subjects is to use a semi-ranking method. I will assume that the subjects are patients, being ranked on intensity of illness from mild to severe. First you pick out a few mild cases and a few severe cases in order to mark the extremes of the range. You then pick out a few cases to form a middle group. You then form another group between the mild and moderate, and another group between moderate and severe. Continue with the rest of the cases putting each patient into his appropriate group. This is done in such a way that, as far as possible, the numbers in the groups are in the proportions of 1, 4, 6, 4 and 1. The members of the groups are then given scores on severity of 1, 2, 3, 4 and 5 respectively. This procedure is repeated at the end of the experiment. Each subject now has two scores, one before treatment and one after and these can be analysed statistically by the usual methods.

So far, I have assumed that you have been comparing two treatments but the techniques can be adapted to comparing three or more treatments. The results can be examined by a special form of analysis of variance, adapted for ranks, known as the Kruskal–Wallis test. The method of ranking can even be adapted to a two-way factorial design. Assuming that one factor consists of several treatments and the other factor is some classification of the subjects then at the end of the experiment, for each level of the second factor, the subjects are ranked for the effects of the treatments. The results are analysed by the Friedman two-way analysis of variance.

Ratings

Another source of difficulty with ranking is that all subjects must be available at the same time for observation and ranking. The method could be used by preparing a written description of each subject or even a video-tape, both before and after treatment, and ranking these, but obviously this is a very clumsy way of doing it. An alternative is to use the method of rating. Whereas in ranking the subjects are compared with each other, in rating methods a series of standards is first devised and then the subjects are ' ranked ' in relation to the standards. This is not really practicable unless the complex pattern to be assessed is subdivided into single variables.

Rating scales have been used chiefly in psychology and psychiatry and they have also been used by social workers for assessing the results of case work. They have been very little used in general medicine and surgery although the first beginnings have been made for thyroid disease, multiple sclerosis and rheumatoid arthritis. The use of multiple criteria is analogous to a rating scale containing many items and I shall consider this later.

The great value of rating scales is that although based on subjective judgements they provide information in a standard form.

This makes it easy to compare subjects with one another, on different occasions, at different centres and by any observer. A second advantage of rating scales is that the information they provide can be easily quantified for statistical analysis.

There are many kinds of rating scale and it is customary to classify them according to their purpose. They can also be classified according to their use by observers or by the subject (self ratings). It is convenient to distinguish between those rating scales which are to be used by skilled, semi-skilled and unskilled observers. Self-ratings by subjects would come under the last heading. It is easy to design rating scales but difficult to design good ones. Even if you don't try to design a rating scale it will be useful to know something about the principles of their construction in order to help you choose a scale suited to your purpose. An invaluable source of information about current scales for use in psychology and psychiatry is to be found in the Mental Measurement Year Books edited by Buros.

Properties of Items

By strict definition, a rating scale is concerned with the categorizing or quantifying of one variable, but it is customary to use the term to describe a set of scales of related variables. Each one is then called an item in the scale. Each item contains a number of defined grades. The simplest type of item contains only two grades: absent or present. This is rarely satisfactory because of the existence of an intermediate state of ' doubtful '. For example, if one asks a patient whether he has ever vomited and he replies that he cannot remember but he thinks he might have done, how does one assess that? When it is not possible to obtain sufficient information to permit of a clear allocation to one of two categories, the opportunity for bias is enormously increased. It is therefore always desirable to convert a dichotomous assessment into one with three grades of absent, doubtful and present.

The third grade can be further improved by dividing it into mild and severe. Further sub-division is possible so that one can end with absent, doubtful, trivial, mild, moderate, severe, very severe and extreme; eight grades in all. In general, the more grades there are the better is the categorization but the difficulty is that with too many the rater cannot decide between them. It is also difficult to define them clearly, and without clear definition of the various grades it is impossible to achieve high reliability.

In recent years there has been a revival of interest in 'analogue' scales. In these, the rater is asked to locate the intensity of the variable by marking a point along a line which runs between the two extremes, i.e. at one end of the line the variable is absent and at the other end it is very severe. This makes for increased flexibility in rating but the increased range of scores that is possible is accompanied by greater difficulty in defining the positions of a rating. Different raters give different values to the points of the line and if the position of the various grades is indicated, then raters tend to locate their assessments on the specified positions. Analogue scales are best used for making overall or global judgements.

The items should be clearly defined, as should also be their grades, and they should be distinct from each other. They should be relevant to the purpose of the scale, because the presence of a number of items which are irrelevant to the current use, makes the scale more difficult to use and decreases its reliability. They should be concerned with attributes which occur frequently in the subjects used. The less frequently they are scored, the less relevant they are for the purpose required. They should cover the required range of the variable and, for the particular type of subject used, should yield an adequate spread of scores. It is of little use if the scores of subjects collect either at one or the other end of the scale because it is difficult then to differentiate between individual subjects.

Use of Rating Scales

Scales should be easy to use and simple to complete and, in the case of scales which are used for rating patients, they should be of such a nature that they do not interfere with the normal practice of clinical work. Obviously, a good scale should have a high reliability and validity and this is one of the first items of information you will want to know when you are choosing a scale. A very long rating scale cannot be completed at the end of an interview, and if it has to be filled in during the interview, it may distract considerably if the rater has continually to keep turning over pages to find particular items.

Raters should be familiar with the attributes they are assessing, and they should also be familiar with the scale they are using. The value of their ratings will be considerably improved if they have had proper training in the use of rating scales and also if they have had some practice in using the scale in the conditions which they will experience during the experiment. The training should be devoted to ensuring that they know how to score items independently and to avoid constant errors. Independent scoring means that any one aspect of behaviour which is included in one item should not be included in another. It also means that when the purpose of a rating is to assess the current state of a subject, the rating should not be influenced by previous ones. It has been demonstrated that when ratings are made on a form on which previous ratings are recorded then they become ' contaminated '. This particular requirement of independence is much more important than is generally realized. To quote Jacobsen, ' Failure to observe this requirement can invalidate months of careful work '.

Raters should be careful not to let their interviews become stereotyped, or degenerate into a set of leading questions. Constant errors are a trap of the unwary. The error of leniency describes a reluctance of the rater to use extreme or severe scores. The halo effect means that the rater tends to give a high score on one variable if he has given high scores on others and vice versa. The logical error is based on a tendency to give high or low scores on different items where these seem sensible or to be implied by the nature of the material. The error of proximity signifies that a rater tends to give similar scores to adjacent items. Central tendency is the commonest of constant errors and refers to the inclination of raters to give middle scores and to be reluctant to move to either end of the scale.

The great criticism which is repeatedly made against the use of ratings is that they are liable to error based upon the subjective state of the rater. It is said that the mood, attitude and patience or impatience of the rater will affect his judgement and so distort the result. I have had many discussions with physicians and surgeons on this point and I have noticed as a matter of empirical experience that the greatest critics of the use of rating methods are those who appear to be most convinced of the accuracy of their diagnoses in clinical practice and of their ability to identify the best applicant for a job when they are serving on selection committees! The criticism is true but only partly so. It is true that by use of appropriate instrumental methods we can decrease the errors of measurement. A grocer does not estimate a pound of sugar with his hands. Although he could learn to do so with an accuracy of less than 5 per cent error, he weighs it on a balance. The reason is simple: we can trust his judgement, but not his bias!

There is little difficulty in reducing the ' errors of measurement ' of ratings to a level as low as we wish. I have already referred briefly to some of the methods that are used. Variables to be judged must be clearly described and the various levels or stages must be properly demarcated. The raters should be trained in their judgement so that they can learn to recognize the sources of bias and diminish them. So much for the factors on the part of the rater. On the other side it is important to ensure that the ratings are done under standard conditions. Thus, patients who suffer from depressive illness often show a characteristic diurnal variation in their symptoms; it would therefore be advisable to do the ratings at the same time of day for each patient. When we try to assess the amount of movement of joints and pain with movement in patients suffering from rheumatoid arthritis, we must ensure that the attitude and mood of the patients is constant each time the observation is made.

The most important method for reducing errors of measurement in subjective ratings is simply replication. You will recollect what I said about the relation between the variance of means and the variance of the parent population; the variance of means is inversely related to the size of the samples. However large the error of measurement may be, as shown by its variance, we can cut it by half by taking two ratings and using the mean of them. We can cut it to a fifth by taking five ratings and using their mean. With this simple method, we can cut it down to any size we wish.

It is customary to say that the many ratings should be made at the same time by different observers. All the raters should be assembled together and should make their judgements simultaneously. Of course, these judgements should be made independently and without collusion or consultation. This makes clear one of the difficulties of the method; it is fairly easy to persuade a colleague to help you with your ratings but when you have to collect three, four or five to come to the one session for carrying out the ratings, then the task is almost impossible. Incidentally, one benefit from simultaneous rating is that, after the ratings have been made, the raters can discuss the reasons for any discrepancies in their assessments, and this helps to standardize the ratings. But for what other reasons should the raters make their assessments at the same time? Why should they not make their judgements on different occasions? The reason is that the subject may have altered from one occasion to another and this will increase the differences between the ratings.

This answer is so simple that it appears to be almost self-evident, but it has important implications which need to be considered carefully.

If the subject varies from one occasion to another, then the measurements that are made, and this is true whatever the method of measurement may be, will also vary. The measurement will have an ' error variance ' arising from the fluctuations in the state of the subject. The error variance of ratings will therefore arise from two sources : one from the differences between raters and the other from the changes in the state of the subject; and you will remember that variances summate. If you and your colleagues have only a limited time available for doing ratings, and you can do, say, only four, then you can do these in two different ways. If you do the ratings simultaneously, you minimize the errors of rating but leave untouched the errors of fluctuation. If you do the ratings at intervals, you minimize the errors of fluctuation and leave untouched the errors of rating. Obviously, the trick is to balance these two so as to reduce the error variance to a minimum. The principle applies equally to instrumental measurements. If you want to measure the temperature of a subject, you may obtain better information by using a simple clinical thermometer several times at suitable intervals and taking the mean of the results, then by using some expensive and elaborate electronic device that will measure accurately to 100th of a degree, but using it only once.

Analysis of Data from Ratings

At the end of your experiment, all the subjects in your different treatment groups will have been rated on a number of variables; they may also have been rated before treatment as well as after. We will consider for the moment the ratings on only one variable. For each group, you count the number of subjects within each grade and thus obtain a frequency distribution. The distributions will differ from one group to another. The null hypothesis states that these frequency distributions do not differ by more than would be obtained by random sampling from the same population and there is a simple statistical test, which I shall describe in due course, to test this hypothesis.

This method of analysing the data makes no assumptions about the relations between the different grades, although the descriptions of the grades imply a quantitative relationship of some sort. Obviously, it would be useful to give some quantitative meaning to the grades and this can be done fairly simply. If the frequency is Gaussian in form then obviously the grades can be assigned to the numbers 0, 1, 2, 3, etc. More accurately, the frequency distributions should correspond to the binomial expansion as illustrated in Lecture 8. For example, if there were five grades, then ideally the frequency distribution should correspond to the ratios of 1, 4, 6, 4 and 1. If they do, then they would be given quantitative form as 0, 1, 2, 3 and 4. Even if, in the population, these grades had relative frequencies in these ratios, sampling error would in general not reproduce the ratios exactly. In practice, therefore, it is sufficient if the frequency distribution is high in the middle grades and lower at the two ends. There is a way of forcing the grades into Gaussian distribution and giving them appropriate quantification scores, but in practice it is not worth doing. A crude quantification like this is enough to make the purist statistician's toes curl with horror, but it works reasonably well in practice. When there are a number of variables to be combined, as is the case with most rating scales, it works extremely well.

Summary

Subjective criteria can be of the greatest importance in clinical investigations. They are liable to various kinds of error but these can be reduced by appropriate methods. The simplest way to use subjective criteria is by the method of ranking. Rating methods are more suitable when the number of subjects is large, and they can be easily quantified. The construction and use of rating scales has been described.

REFERENCES

BUROS, O. K. (1968). *The Sixth Mental Measurements Year Book.* New Brunswick: Rutger's University Press.

JACOBSEN, M. (1965). The use of rating scales in clinical research. *British Journal of Psychiatry,* **111,** 545-546.

LANE, P. & WILLIAMSON, D. M. (1969). Treatment of acne vulgaris with Tetracycline Hydrochloride: a double-blind trial with 51 patients. *British Medical Journal,* **i,** 76-79.

Prediction and Measure of Association

Very often in clinical medicine, we may need information about some variable which is too difficult to obtain in routine clinical practice. In such cases, we often measure another variable, because it will give us a figure which is closely related to the one we want. Thus we use a sphygmomanometer to measure ' blood pressure ', instead of using an intra-arterial catheter. The actual measurement is not quite the same but it is near enough. Sometimes what we measure is quite different from what we want to measure, but since it increases and decreases in the same way, it may suffice for our purposes. Such a test is the routine estimation of sugar in the urine instead of the blood, for keeping check on the control of diabetes. There is another measurement which we would commonly like to make or know, but it is not possible to do so because it is not yet available, and that is the amount of recovery of a patient after treatment. Predicting the results of treatment and estimating one variable from another are formally the same.

Covariance and Correlation

When we make a measurement on a subject, we obtain some information about him. Previously we had no information, now we have some. A statistician would point out that if we knew that the subject was a member of a particular population, then we would have some information about him, and on this basis we could guess what value the measurement would be. For example, if I ask you to guess the weight of a man, knowing only that he is an adult, then your best guess is the population mean, which is about 73 kilograms. The reason why this is the best guess is that, in the long run, the average of your guesses (always the mean) will equal the population mean. Furthermore it can be proved that you will be less wrong by guessing this particular figure than by using any other one.

If I then tell you that he is well above average in height, you might guess that he was, say, 77 kilos in weight. If I said that he was obviously shorter than the average, you would guess that he was about 68 kilos in weight. These guesses would be more accurate than the original guess because you would now have some information about the individual. This information rests on the fact that in the population as a whole, taller men are heavier than the average and shorter men lighter; height and weight co-vary in the population. If we describe this co-variance in quantitative terms, then we can use a measurement on one variable to estimate the measurement on the other. This will become clear if we consider an actual example before going on further. Table 13.1 gives the distribution of patients according to their age and length of stay in hospital.

TABLE 13.1

Distribution of 126 patients according to age and stay in hospital

		Age in years							
		<30	30–34	35–39	40–44	45–49	50–54	>54	Total
	31–35						2	5	7
	26–30					4	7	12	23
Length of	21–25				6	3	3	1	13
stay in	16–20		2	1	8	11	8	2	32
years	11–15	1	3	3	7	6	5	1	26
	6–10	3	3	4	3	6	1		20
	<6	3		1	1				5
	Total	7	8	9	25	30	26	21	126

If we are looking through hospital records, and for some reason the patient's age is missing, then the best estimate we can make for his age is to assume that he is between 45 and 49 years old. From the above table, it can be seen that in this way we are more likely to be right than if we choose any other age. If, however, we know that he has been in hospital less than six years, the best guess for his age would be that he is under 30 years. If he has been in 26 to 30 years, the best guess is that he is over 54, and so on. Without any information about the patient, we choose that figure which will make us correct as often as possible, but even this will be right less than one in four times. With some information, we can improve our estimates and be correct in a larger proportion of cases. Now let us look at Table 13.2.

We can see that the commonest score for 'behaviour in the ward' is between 30 to 39, and in the absence of any information about a patient, this is the best estimate we can make of what his score is likely to be. If we know his age, this will not enable us to make a better estimate. In two columns the most frequent score is between 10 and 19, in two others between 20 and 29 and in three between 30 and 39. The largest figures in the columns do not differ much from the others and their positions do not show any trend. Whatever the age, the commonest score tends to be roughly between 20 and 39. These are tables actually obtained during the course of an investigation on the effects of treatment on chronic patients in a mental hospital. As such, they therefore lack the neatness and clarity of artificial tables, but I hope that they are all the more convincing for that reason.

TABLE 13.2

Distribution of 126 patients according to age and behaviour-score

| | | Age | | | | | | | |
		<30	30–34	35–39	40–44	45–49	50–54	>54	Total
	60–69				1				1
	50–59		2	1	3	2	1	2	11
	40–49		1	1	2	6	3	4	17
Score for	30–39	2	2	3	5	8	5	5	30
behaviour	20–29	1	1	1	7	3	6	7	26
in ward	10–19	3	1	2	5	7	9	2	29
	0–9	1	1	1	2	4	2	1	12
	Total	7	8	9	25	30	26	21	126

In order to estimate the magnitude of one variable from the measurement of an associated variable, it is necessary to calculate a 'regression equation'. When both variables are measured as deviations from their means and in standard measure, i.e. the deviation is divided by the standard deviation, the regression equation is in the form $y = b \cdot x$, where y is being estimated from the known score of x. In that equation, b is a number ranging from $+1$, which gives perfect estimation, down to zero which gives none, and down to -1 which again gives perfect estimation but indicates that as one variable increases the other decreases.

If you consider this equation carefully, you will see that the estimated deviation of y from its mean is in the form of a fraction (weight less than 1) of the deviation of x from its mean. This may seem excessively simple, if not even simple minded. Surely, y could be related to x squared or x cubed or some other function of x. The answer is that by some appropriate 'transformation' of the variables we can usually reduce the equation to the simple form. For example, if $y=x^3$ then by taking logarithms we change the equation to log y=3 log x and this is in the same form as before. Some ingenuity may be required to find a suitable transformation, and if the worse comes to the worst, it will be sufficient to find some approximation.

In the equation y=b·x, the b is known as a 'regression co-efficient', but it is more usual to consider it as a 'correlation coefficient', which indicates the relationship between the two variables. When the correlation is zero, we know that information about one variable does not give information about the second one. This is shown very clearly in the regression equation, because when the b is zero, then whatever the x may be, the resulting y will always be zero. Since we are measuring in the form of deviations from the mean, the score of zero signifies that we are at the mean, and you will remember that that is exactly what we estimate in the absence of any information apart from membership of the popu-lation.

A correlation coefficient describes the relationship between two variables and once one has become accustomed to that sort of measure, it is very useful for compressing a good deal of data into a compact and informative shape. For experimental purposes, it is generally better to think of a correlation coefficient in terms of a regression coefficient, for estimating or 'predicting' one variable from another. In the population or sample, prediction is perfect when the coefficient is 1, which means that, given the measure x for a particular individual, we can tell exactly what his y will be. When the correlation is less than 1, then our prediction is less accurate and we can only estimate roughly what the value of y will be. In general, the actual y will differ from the predicted y, it will be either greater or lesser. If we subtract the predicted y from the actual y, we shall have a set of deviations from prediction and we can calculate their variance.

This variance is of the greatest importance. Take the case when the regression coefficient is zero. For each individual in the group, the 'predicted' y is the group mean. We take the predicted y score, subtract it from the actual y. We square all the deviations, sum them and divide by the degrees of freedom. We now have the variance of deviation from prediction; but this is exactly how we calculate the variance of the original y scores. Now take the case where the regression coefficient is 1. The predicted y now exactly equals the obtained y, the deviations are zero and so is their variance. Between regression coefficients of 0 and 1, the variance of deviation from prediction ranges between the variance of y to zero. Thus the variance of y has been divided into two portions, the variance of prediction, i.e. that portion accounted for by the variation in x, and the variance of deviation from prediction or residual variance.

Let us see now how we can apply this to a clinical investigation. We will suppose that we wish to compare the effect of two different drugs in reducing blood cholesterol. We plan the experiment in the usual way and measure the blood cholesterol before and after treatment in two groups of subjects given the two treatments. The cholesterol levels after treatment will reflect the efficacy of the treatment and can be compared in the usual way; but they will also be related to the original levels before treatment. As I mentioned in the previous lecture we can tackle this by analysing the experiment as a factorial design, one factor being the two treatments and the other factor being the initial concentration of cholesterol divided into high, medium and low. We can, however, analyse the results in a different way. We start by assuming that there is no difference in the effects of the two treatments. We then take the initial levels and final levels after treatment for each subject and we calculate a regression equation and predict what the final level will be from the individual's initial level. If we then find that in the group given one treatment, the actual levels are consistently below those predicted (and in the other group they are consistently above) we have then demonstrated that one treatment is more effective than the other.

This is a very laborious way of carrying out the calculation and the usual procedure is much simpler. The usual statistical test divides the total variance of the criterion scores (final cholesterol levels, Y scores) into that between groups and that within groups. The latter is the variance of Y, independent of the differences between the groups. The next step is to calculate the variance due to prediction or, as it is usually called, the variance due to regression and subtract it from the within-group variance. Finally, the between-groups variance is divided by the residual variance to give the F ratio. It is obvious that the F ratio will now be larger and its statistical significance therefore greater. The analysis of covariance has therefore increased the sensitivity of the experiment to detect the effects of the experimental treatments, and in this lies its great value.

Multiple Correlation

As I have mentioned, it would be extremely useful in many circumstances to know how well a patient would respond to treatment. Usually we have a fair idea of this, but such ideas are based on the known outcome for certain categories of patients, and we assume that this will apply to the particular patient, provided we can subsume him under the appropriate categories. For instance, we may know that old patients will do badly, and young ones better; that acute onset of illness is more favourable than a slow onset, and so on. The clinician classifies the patient according to the various categories and then tries to counterbalance the favourable against the unfavourable indications and arrive at some sort of conclusion. In an undefined way, these favourable and unfavourable factors are summed (added and subtracted) in the physician's mind to make some sort of total. The result is generally given in general terms such as the chances are bad, good or excellent.

It is possible to do this very much more precisely by means of an extension of the notion of correlation. Let us assume for the moment that the outcome of treatment has been quantified, i.e. stated in the form of some sort of figure which is a measure of the patient's condition. We can then investigate a number of variables, which can be measured before the patient receives his treatment, and then correlate them with the result of the treatment. When we have sufficient cases measured and followed-up (and the number increases rapidly with the increase in the number of variables we measure before treatment) we can then use the variable with the biggest correlation to give us a prediction of outcome. We can go further: we can use the information from the other variables to increase the size of our correlation and therefore improve the prediction. This is done by the method of multiple correlation. The process of calculating a multiple correlation is complicated, but the final result gives us a regression equation in which the different variables are added up, each with an appropriate weighting, to give an estimate of the outcome of treatment, i.e. give a figure which is a measure of the outcome.

Few attempts have been made to use multiple correlation for this purpose in clinical medicine. partly because the use of these techniques is still very new in this field, but also because there is not often much point in it. After all, in most cases, a patient can expect not to be *worse* after treatment, and he is likely to be better. So even if the amount of improvement is not likely to be large, it will still be worth his while to accept the treatment offered. Nevertheless, when the treatment may be dangerous, take up much time, be extremely unpleasant or even very expensive, it might be worthwhile for the physician and patient to have as good an idea as is possible of what is to be expected. In such circumstances, the use of multiple correlation could be of great value.

I have emphasized that multiple correlation is used when all the variables can be measured, i.e. are quantifiable. This is not entirely true, for it can be used when some of the variables, or even all, are qualitative. Examples of such qualitative variables are sex, blood group, eye colour, before or after puberty or the menopause, positive or negative Mantoux test, and even being with or without an appendix! The most interesting of the extensions of multiple correlation is that in which the criterion to be predicted is qualitative and not quantitative. Examples of such are recovery or not, discharge from hospital or not, retention in the armed forces or discharge, and so on. The regression formula which 'predicts' qualitative categories which are mutually exclusive is known as a 'discriminant function', and it can be used for 'predicting', or rather, allocating an individual, not only to one of two mutually exclusive categories, but to one of several. In recent years there have been a number of attempts to use discriminant functions to help in another activity which is apparently very unlike what I have been talking about, but which formally is the same, and that is, the making of a diagnosis.

When a physician makes a diagnosis, he takes a history, makes a clinical examination and supplements this, when necessary, by physical and chemical investigations. He assembles all this data, some of which is in quantitative form, but much of which is qualitative, assembles it in his mind and from the result, he allocates the patient to a particular diagnostic category. Such diagnostic categories are, in general, qualitatively different and mutually exclusive. Under certain limited conditions, it has been shown that this can be done very simply and very efficiently by means of the calculation of a discriminant function. The best examples have been in the diagnosis of thyroid disease.

Although, in the case of disease of the thyroid, diagnosis is essentially a dichotomous classification, i.e. the patient is allocated to one of two mutually exclusive categories: 'normal' or 'suffering from disease' (hypo- or hyperthyroidism, depending on the type of symptoms considered), in general, the process of making a diagnosis consists of allocating a patient to one of very many possibilities, and this is precisely what the technique of multiple discriminant functions does; though it is not yet applicable to the general problems of making a diagnosis. In a few conditions, a number of alternative treatments are available, for example, several drugs as well as electroshock, are available for the treatment of depressive states, and the number of hypotensive drugs is now so great that I long ago lost count. In surgery, alternative operative procedures are sometimes available, e.g. gastric operations. The use of multiple discriminant technique could make a real contribution to the problem of clarifying the indications for the use of a particular treatment and the first attempts have already been made.

Multiple Measurements

In giving an account of various types of experiment, I have always assumed that the criterion of improvement could be described in terms of one variable, for example, a decrease in blood pressure, or an increase in weight. Where the criterion is essentially qualitative, I have assumed that it was handled by dichotomy : recovered or not, alive or dead. These two types of criterion are not always applicable or informative. Sometimes improvement is a much more subtle phenomenon, and the use of some single measurement is obviously unsatisfactory.

We can divide 'improvement' into its separate variables, and consider each of them separately. At first sight it would then appear simple to do a test of statistical significance on each variable, but it is immediately obvious that the results might appear confusing, for one could imagine a situation in which one variable gave a significant result, and another did not. How does one interpret that? There are other difficulties which are much more important. The more measurements that are made, the more certain is it that some are going to be 'significant' by chance alone. This is a risk that is taken with every experiment, but multiple measurements obviously increase the risk. Finally, the fact that the different measurements are all aspects of what one means by 'improvement' makes it very likely that they are correlated, i.e. as one improves the others will tend to do so. Since the variables are not independent, the tests of significance are not independent, so that if one is ' significant ', the others will tend to be ' significant ' too. This appears to contradict what I have just said, that the test may speak with different voices, but I am speaking of tendencies only. The real difficulty is that the use of additional variables, because of the correlation between them, does not necessarily increase our information very much.

There are appropriate statistical techniques for dealing with multiple measurements, and these form that branch of statistics known as ' multivariate analysis '. These correspond with the univariate tests that I have already described. When we compare several treatments, using a single criterion, we then examine the results by the analysis of variance with its ' F ratio '; when the criterion is multiple, we use multivariate analysis of variance with its corresponding ' lambda ratio '. Multivariate statistical tests have been little used in the past, as they are impracticable without computers.

Let me illustrate this with an example based on an investigation actually made. Suppose you want to compare two treatments for polyarthritis. You would have little difficulty in setting up the experiment, but what would you use as criterion for improvement? Increase in the range of movement of a joint? Yes, but which joint? You might try some overall measure of improvement such as strength in grip of the hands, or time taken to walk a measured distance. It is obvious that no single one can have precedence over the others, or be considered adequate to represent the others, without setting up a preliminary investigation to settle this question. Such an investigation would take a long time and would require many, many patients. Meanwhile, there is still the practical problem presented by the new treatment. In such a situation, the easiest way out would be to make all the measurements on the patients and then use them all in one single test of statistical significance.

I don't want to suggest that all problems can be solved in this way. There is not much difficulty about the statistical problems: the tests are available, and provided that the data are suitable, the tests can be done. The real problems are quite different, and I am sure that you will not be surprised to hear that they are clinical. These complex statistical tests are not easy to interpret clinically and there is little doubt that their application to clinical medicine is going to raise many problems. But then, who thought that clinical medicine was simple?

There is, however, a simple way of combining a number of criteria into a single index of change, but the problem arises of how to combine them. For example, they may be measured in milligrammes, microgrammes, 'units' and milliequivalents, and these cannot be summed as such. The way in which it is done is as follows. (It is important that all the measures should be available for every patient.) All the measures are first converted into standard units, i.e. the mean and standard deviation of each of the measures is calculated, then each measure is converted to a deviation from the mean, by subtracting the mean from it, and then each deviation is divided by the standard deviation. The standard scores are then summed as they are, which means that each one is given a weight of $+1$. Sometimes it will be found that improvement is related to an increase in a measurement and to a decrease in another. When that is so, the measures that show a decrease should be given a weighting of -1, i.e. they are subtracted from the total. This may seem peculiar at first sight, but if we consider the case of a patient who improves and measure X increases, but measure Y decreases, then, when we measure the changes as deviations, X becomes, say, $+x$, and Y becomes $-y$. When the Y variable is given a negative weighting, this means that the index will be $x+y$. To give all the variables the same weight is rather a crude method, though surprisingly effective in practice. Strictly speaking, one should take into account the correlations between the variables, but it does not make much difference if we do not.

The resemblance of this procedure to the adding up of the scores on the items of a rating scale is obvious. In the case of a rating scale, it is unnecessary to convert the scores on the items into standard form because the items are scored in 'units' anyway and, even more important, the ranges and standard deviations of the items are approximately the same. When we sum the crude scores, the weights (in standard form) are not the same as the weights of $+1$ which we would give to the standardized scores, but the difference is small; and the more items we sum together to form a total score, the less important is the difference in the weights.

It is sometimes argued that to add together variables which are qualitatively different produces a sum which is meaningless; chalk and cheese cannot be added together to give any meaningful total. Such objections are due to a misunderstanding of the meaning of such a total score. It is not possible for me to give here an exact description of the circumstances under which such a summation is justifiable and meaningful; but ignoring certain qualifications, it can be said that the change or improvement which we are measuring is a complex phenomenon and each of the variables which we measure can be regarded as one aspect of it. We can therefore regard each variable as an inaccurate measure of the total. When we have a number of inaccurate measures, we can improve our accuracy by taking their mean, which is equivalent to taking their sum.

Standard Scores in Clinical Practice

At this point, I would like to step aside from the consideration of pure research problems and give you an example of how ideas used in research can have direct clinical value. We make many measurements in clinical practice and sometimes, though not always, we need to know the full details of the measurement in order to take appropriate action. This happens when we wish to replace deficient constituents of the blood, for example, the total volume, potassium or sodium. On most occasions, however, such as in making a diagnosis or monitoring response to treatments, it is sufficient to know the relative position of the individual patient, either in relation to his previous state or to the population as a whole. In the latter case, we are trying to decide whether the measurements we obtain signify that the patient's function is normal, or abnormal due to disease. Since it is impossible to remember the norms of all the tests that are used on patients, it is customary for laboratories to provide a range of scores that are to be found in normals. This is helpful but it is not enough. When a given test-result is well within or well outside the limits given it is easy to interpret, but when it is within a few points of these limits (in terms of the units of measurement) it is very difficult to interpret. In order to do so, we should know what sort of measurements we would obtain from normal subjects and this means knowing the distribution of these measurements. In other words, we have to know the mean and standard deviation. On this basis we can determine the probability that the patient comes from a normal or healthy population. Similarly, if we know the mean and standard deviation of the measurement to be found in patients who show abnormal function, arising from different disorders, we can determine the probability that a patient comes from the various abnormal populations. This is much better than a 'normal range', but we would still have to remember the mean and standard deviation of every test.

I have just pointed out that if you wish to combine a number of criteria into a single index you have first to convert them to standard form. A standard score is such that the population mean is zero and the standard deviation is 1, and if the distribution of such scores is of Gaussian form then we can also ascertain probabilities by looking up the tables. Thus a standard score of 1·0 and over is found in 15·9 per cent of the population, a standard score of 2·0 and over is obtained with a frequency of 2·3 per cent, and of 2·5 and over in 0·6 per cent of the population.

Let us consider what a transformation into standard scores achieves. The original variables may have been haemoglobin, measured in grams per 100 ml of blood, bilirubin measured in milligrams per 100 ml of plasma, alkaline phosphatase measured in units per 100 ml of plasma and sodium measured as milliequivalents per litre of blood. All these have been changed into one unit of measurement which, when we have become accustomed to it, is perfectly easy to interpret. The distribution may be such that it is necessary to transform the scores, e.g. taking log scores, but in most cases the 'normalizing' of the distribution and obtaining standard scores can be carried out in one procedure. If standard scores were to come into general use, it would enormously simplify the investigation of patients. The physician would order a series of tests and these would be returned from the laboratory all measured in one unit. At a glance, he could tell whether the results were normal, obviously abnormal, or somewhere in between.

A further refinement would be to convert the standard scores into T-score form. This is done by multiplying the standard scores by ten, which gives a standard deviation of 10, and then adding 50 to give a mean of 50. The first step eliminates the need for decimal fractions, because whole numbers (integers) are accurate to a tenth of a standard deviation, and this is sufficient for all practical purposes. The second step eliminates negative scores because they will occur less than three times in a million. If all test results were transformed into T-score form, we would know that the mean of the population was 50 (i.e. of the relevant population; it might be necessary to use different transformations for men and women). Scores between 30 and 70 would be found in 95 per cent of the normal population and could be regarded as normal; scores between 20 and 30, and between 70 and 80 would be suspect, and scores below 20 and above 80 could be accepted as definitely abnormal. This would apply not only to all tests in current use but also to all tests which will ever be devised. It will come about one day and then physicians will wonder how on earth we were able to cope with the present-day chaos.

Summary

Covariance and correlation express the relationship between two variables in mathematical form. An account has been given of their application to clinical experimentation and to the problems raised by the use of multiple variables. They are of fundamental importance in prediction, e.g. results of treatment and also for classification. Examples of the latter in clinical work are the making of a diagnosis and the selection of an appropriate treatment. The information from many variables can be combined by converting the original measurements into standard scores. Such scores could bring about an immense simplification in the interpretation of clinical tests.

REFERENCES

HAMILTON, M. (1958). Measurement in medicine. *Lancet,* **i,** 977-982.
HAMILTON, M. (1969). *New Scientist,* **2, 4,** 504-505.
McGUIRE, R. J. & WRIGHT, V. (1971). A statistical approach to indices of disease activity in rheumatoid arthritis, with reference to a trial of Indomethacin. *Annals of the Rheumatic Diseases,* **30,** 574-580.

Preparation of Data

To undertake good research, it is necessary to know the principles of experimentation but this is insufficient without the knowledge of how to apply them. Lack of organization and mistakes about practical problems can eventually end in chaos and loss of data. In this lecture, I am going to deal with practical aspects of organization and to say a few words on the writing up of results. Some of these details I learned from experienced research workers and others I learned the hard way. I did not realize the importance of these small points until I found myself in the position of trying to help beginners. Attention to these matters will make your work go smoothly; neglect of them will soon land you in an inextricable mess.

Data

You must decide at the beginning what information you want to collect, and then make your trial run. The experience you gain will enable you to revise your decisions on what you need for your investigation and what you can safely ignore. It may be that in follow-up and prospective enquiries you may find, as you go along, that you will need information on additional matters, and some of the data collected may appear to be of little value. Add the new material but continue with the old items until you have a sufficient number of subjects to enable you to analyse the data that you now think are unnecessary. Only then, having found good evidence that they are unwanted, may you abandon items.

It is always difficult to decide how much information to collect and it is only too easy to obscure your investigation with a clutter of useless information. On the one hand, it is not easy to obtain a sufficient number of subjects; planning and preparing a clinical investigation takes a long time; the investigation itself will not be completed until many months have passed; all these are very good reasons for collecting as much information about the subjects as possible while one is about it. On the other hand, collecting a lot of information from each subject does take much time and effort; it is easy to become lost amidst a vast mass of data; a statistical analysis of many items of information takes a long time and seems to lead nowhere; all these are good reasons for not collecting more information than is necessary. It is difficult to come to a wise decision, but you will find it a useful guide to consider always the relevance of the information to your problem. Remember, that a planned programme of research is not undertaken merely to satisfy idle curiosity. Consider therefore the sort of results you will obtain, i.e. all the different possible answers. What inferences could be drawn from these answers, and what sort of light will they cast on your main problem? You will then be able to make clear decisions which time will confirm.

Forms

When you record the information about your subjects, do not rely on hospital and other records. You should design forms on which to record your information and you will probably need a number of different forms for each subject. My experience is that it is useful to have a form for general information about the subject, another to describe his condition at the start of the investigation, and special forms for intermediate and final assessments to record the effects of treatment, but I am not suggesting that this is always necessary. For subjective judgements, you should use a separate copy of a form every time you make an assessment. Assessments should be made without reference to the previous ones so as to ensure that they are not influenced by them. This is not a purely theoretical point as it has been demonstrated in practice, as I pointed out in Lecture 12, that the effects of a treatment can be obscured if assessments are biased by knowledge of previous ones. This is not the method in clinical practice, but it is necessary in research because measurements should be independent; that is the basis of the statistical analysis.

Forms should be filled in at the time the information is obtained. If you put this off until later, you will forget the information or forget to fill in the form. When you have completed a form, always check it so see that it is complete. It may be that some item has been omitted because you did not have the information available. If that is so, you should keep a special note-book on which to record the fact that an item is missing, and make a point of getting the necessary information as soon as possible. Put it into the form first, and then cross out the note in your book. Make a habit of going over your forms to ensure that they have been completed and can be safely stored away. It is surprising how often you will find items missing, often quite simple ones, such as the name or number of the patient, the date when the form was filled, and so on. Again and again I hear clinicians express surprise at the incompleteness of routine hospital records, when they try to do retrospective inquiries. My own experience, and that of most clinical research workers, is that even when every attempt is made to record full information, it is extraordinarily difficult to do so. As a result I tend to be surprised how much information is available in routine records since my expectations are very low!

You should expend some thought and care on the design of your forms. It is very important that they should be easy to read, not only at the time when they are filled in, but subsequently. It is very useful to arrange them so that the required information forms a column, or perhaps two columns. A form in which the data is scattered all over the sheet in the middle of printed matter and instructions, is very difficult to read, and this means that when it is copied or the data extracted, it will be very easy to make mistakes. Figure 14.1 illustrates a form which is badly designed in this way. When the same item appears on several forms, try to put them in the same place on each form. This applies particularly to identifying information, which should be on every form. It can be very exasperating when the name and code number of a patient is in one corner on one form

CASE NO:

DEPRESSED MOOD	
0	Absent
1	Feels low in spirits
2	Feels low. Weeps
3	Frequent weeping Feels helpless
4	Beyond weeping Feels hopeless

HYPOCHONDRIASIS	
0	Absent
1	Preoccupations with bodily functions
2	Fear of physical illness
3	Conviction of physical illness
4	Delusions of bodily change

ANXIETY (Psychic)	
0	Absent
1	Slight
2	Moderate
3	Severe
4	Very severe

DRYNESS OF MOUTH	
0	Absent
1	Trivial
2	Moderate
3	Marked

DIURNAL VARIATION OF MOOD
Absent
Worse in morning
Worse in afternoon
Worse in evening

Figure 14.1. Unsatisfactory lay-out for forms.

and another corner on another. Identifying data should be 'redundant'; you should include the case-number, name age, sex, marital status, perhaps even the address, and also the date. Otherwise you may find yourself trying to disentangle the forms of two subjects named J. Smith, age 35 years. Figure 14.2 illustrates an improved lay-out.

INSTRUCTIONS AND CODING

You should prepare a special sheet of instructions on how to fill in each form. The instructions should mention every item. This may seem unnecessary, but if you are working with collaborators, you will find that it is. It can easily happen that one person fills in the length of history in months and the other in years. One gives the age last birthday and the other at the next birthday, and so on. Some people like to have the instructions printed on the form itself, but I prefer to have them on a separate sheet. When you come to look at the data, it is much easier if the sheet is not cluttered up with instructions; it is also less bulky and therefore easier to handle. I cannot repeat this too often: a clear form is easy to read and so you make less mistakes. It is also easier to fill in and it takes less time. This is important, because you are usually doing this in the course of an interview, and you need your time and concentration for that.

NAME: .... AGE: ...... SEX: ...... DATE: .... CASE No: ....

SYMPTOMS	RANGE	SCORE
1. Depression	0 - 4	
2. Anxiety	0 - 4	
3 Hypochondriasis	0 - 4	
4. Dryness of mouth	0 - 3	
5. Diurnal Variation M (ring which one) A E	0 - 2	

Assessor's Initials

Figure 14.2. Improved lay-out for forms.

For convenience in analysing the data, it is customary to put all data into coded form, and this is always in the form of numbers. For example, sex will be recorded eventually as 1 for females and 0 for males (or vice versa). This coding is used for all dichotomous data, e.g. previous medical or surgical treatment, slow or sudden onset, family history present or absent. If several treatments are available (when recording previous attacks of the illness) then list them all and give each one a number. Even when data are already in numerical form, it is often convenient to substitute a simple number for the original figures. Thus age might be recorded in decades, and 0 to 9 years recorded as 0, 10 to 19 recorded as 1, 20 to 29 years as 2 and so on. The same could be done for red-cell count, blood-sugar concentration, etc. Sometimes it is convenient to subtract a constant figure from the actual figure, e.g. you could deduct 40 kilos from the weight of your patients, or 100 cm from the height. You could divide a red-cell count by 100,000 to give a two-digit number. It is unnecessary to record empirical measurements with more than two significant digits; even that implies an accuracy of measurement of 1 per cent.

The coding of data can be done at the time when the form is filled in, but unless you have had plenty of practice with the coding, it is better to leave it until later. You can also decide to put the coded information on the original form, but this may be very inconvenient, in which case it should be left until a later stage.

Assembling the Data

Sooner or later, you will have finished with a particular subject, and you will then have a number of forms for him. These forms should be pinned together, but they should not be stapled permanently until you have finished with them and can put them away. Such a set of forms is very inconvenient to handle, so the next stage is to assemble all the information found on the various forms on to one sheet. It is at this stage that it is most convenient to code the data. I have mentioned that it is very useful to have a special form for general information about the subject, and this form could be used for recording all the subseqent information about him. This may not be practicable, for there may not be enough room on it. I also use this form for the case history of patients, which is put down in the usual narrative form. If you should want to refresh your memory about a particular patient, or you want to give some illustrative case-histories, it is a great convenience to have the material available on your forms, and not to have to search in the hospital records for what you want.

You started off with a number of forms for each subject and then assembled the data so that you have one form for each patient. The next stage is to prepare a master sheet. This will contain all the information for all your subjects. You could prepare the master sheet from the original set of forms, and this eliminates a second copying with its risks of errors, but it may be inconvenient if the coding has to be done at the same time. You may have to have several master sheets if you have many subjects, in which case it may be convenient to classify them and have a separate sheet for each group, e.g. one sheet for men and one for women. If you can leave this task until the end of the investigation, you could use a separate sheet for each treatment but it is better to fill in the master sheet as you go along. At the top of the sheet you put down headings for each item of information, and down the left-hand side you put the subjects' case numbers (or names). Incidentally, it is a useful trick to use the case numbers for classifying your subjects. Thus case numbers 0 to 99 could be used for males and 100 to 199 for females. Case numbers 0 to 49 could be used for one centre and and 50 to 99 for another. The data for each subject are then inserted, in coded form, along a row. In this way all the data of the trial is visible in compact form suitable for study. The separate items are in columns, which are easy to total. The rows, which represent patients, should also be totalled, and obviously the sums of the rows and the columns should be equal. This serves as a check of the arithmetic. The totals of the columns are then divided by the number of patients, and the averages entered at the bottom of each column. It is now easy to compare the different groups.

The master sheet has another function, for it can be handed in for punching the data on to cards. The usual arrangement is for all the data for one patient to be punched on to one card. Once this has been done, much of the labour of calculation can be eliminated. The most tedious part of statistical calculations is the calculation of sums and sums of squares, and this is very easily done by machine. Of course, if you have access to a computer, it will be able to do all your statistical analysis.

PUNCHED CARDS

Punched cards are of two types: for hand punching or machine punching. In the U.K. the former go by the name of Paramount and Findex. In the Paramount system, the cards are already punched with holes around the edge and information is recorded on the card by converting a hole into a slot by means of a pair of clippers. See Figure 14.3. This is particularly suitable for dichotomous data, e.g. one treatment is clipped as a slot and the other as a hole. The cards are used primarily for sorting and this is done as follows: The cards are assembled into a neat pack, and a long needle is inserted into the appropriate hole. The pack is then lifted and gently tapped and shaken, whereupon all the cards that have a slot at that point fall down, can be separated and counted. By appropriate coding methods you can sort the subjects into any combination of categories and even find the card for a particular subject.

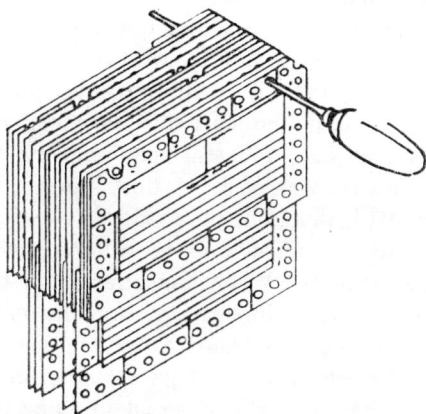

Figure 14.3. Edge-punched cards—Paramount. (By courtesy of Copeland Chatterson Co. Ltd., Seymour House, 17 Waterloo Place, London, SW1 4AR.)

This method is particularly useful when subjects accumulate slowly. Since only a minimum of apparatus is required for handling the cards, they can be used when no other facilities are available. As each subject arrives, the card is prepared for him. The data can also be written out on the card, which can be obtained suitably printed to serve as a form. The system is simple, easy to use and cheap, but it becomes clumsy when the number of subjects is large. If you are going to have more than 50, it is better to use machine-punched cards.

The Findex system has holes punched all over the card, and a special device is used to punch the hole into a slot. Another special device has to be used for sorting the cards. Its only advantage is that much more information can be punched on it. Findex cards are very little used in research.

Machine-punched cards have 80 columns and each column has ten positions for the digits 0 to 9 and two others, the x and y positions, for other kinds of information, e.g. a minus sign. To record a number, a rectangular hole is punched in the appropriate place in a column. See Figure 14.5. Two-digit numbers are punched in two adjacent columns. A set of columns used for recording a multi-digit number is known as a ' field '. There is no need to learn how to punch the cards yourself as there are many firms who will do it quite cheaply. When you go to have your cards punched, it will be necessary for you to take your master sheets with you and explain exactly what you want to have done. There will be no difficulty with this if you have written out your master sheets neatly. If your cards are going to be dealt with by a computer, it will be necessary for you to find out exactly how they should be punched. This should be done at the start of your investigation. Different computer programs have different requirements; for example, if one of your items consists of a two-digit number, then some programs require that it should be punched as a two-digit number even if the value is less than ten, thus 17 will be punched as 17 and 7 will be punched as 07. When you arrange for the punching of your data, always order a duplicate pack. Sometimes cards become bent or even torn and it is handy to have a spare one available. Data can also be punched on to paper tape, for reading into a computer (Fig. 14.4). There is no point in going into the relative merits of punched cards or tape. Although computers can read both kinds, in practice most computer installations tend to use only one or the other and you will probably have no choice.

When the tape or cards are punched, you will hand them in to the computer installation and in due course, if all goes well, the result will be handed back to you. This seems to be the answer to the clinician's prayers, but I am afraid that it is not quite so. In the first place, in order to have all the computing done for you, you must know precisely what you want to have done and be able to give the necessary instructions. You will never really learn this until you have done some computing yourself. In the second place, you must prepare yourself for delay and frustration. Your data will have to be prepared to conform exactly with the requirements of the programs and even the most trivial of discrepancies will block the computing. It may take hours of work to find out what is wrong, and even experienced workers may be baffled. Punched cards may be rejected for no apparent reason; paper-tape copiers cannot be trusted to copy 20 metres of tape without making errors; all sorts

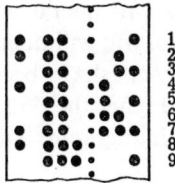

Figure 14.4. Section of punched paper tape. (Reproduced from ALGOL ICL Student Edition, by permission of International Computers Ltd.)

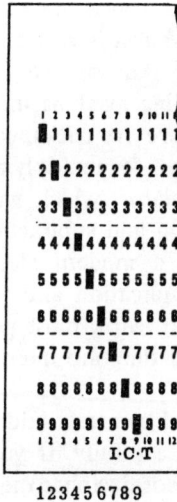

Part of a punched card

Figure 14.5. Part of a punched card. (Reproduced from ALGOL ICL Student Edition, by permission of International Computers Ltd.)

of things may go wrong unexpectedly. It is a safe rule that you should never arrange to have computing done against a deadline. If you can have access to a modern electronic desk calculating machine then, unless the task is quite impracticable, it will usually be worth your while doing your own computing. Surprising as it

7

may seem to you, once you have got over the drudgery of calculating sums and sums of squares, the actual work involved in doing the tests of significance is really quite interesting, and it is very exciting to see the results coming out.

What is much more important is that data should be looked at carefully. In this way you will obtain a grasp of what has been happening and, furthermore, you will obtain ideas for further work. As my experience has grown, I have become more and more impressed by the value of studying the data. Sort out your data and study them. Plot them out into graphs. This is hard and slow work, but it will repay every effort.

COMPUTING

If you do not have any access to machine facilities, you will have to do your own computing. At the worst, you can do everything you want with paper and pencil, aided by tables of logarithms, squares and square roots; but it is very rare to find yourself in such an unfortunate situation. Almost every organization except the smallest will have an adding machine in some office, and this will save you much work. There are tricks, easily learned, whereby an adding machine can be used for multiplying. Most accounts departments have a desk calculator, which will do multiplication and division as well as addition and subtraction. If you are lucky, you will find that they have a modern electrical machine that will also do cumulative multiplication and automatic squaring. Such machines are very easy to learn, most people become adept with them in half an hour and they are interesting toys with which to play.

Your calculations should be neatly laid out on the paper and you should write your figures carefully. If you don't, you will be surprised how often you cannot decipher the numbers. The digits 3, 5 and 8 can look remarkably alike, and so can 6, 9 and 0. This is even more important when you are writing out your master sheet if it is to be read by a card-punch operator. Describe in words each stage of the computing and label each sheet very carefully. It is a useful trick to put the date down too. I assure you that it is a very disconcerting experience to find a sheet of figures and not be able to identify them. Use good paper, all of one size: I have a bad habit of using any handy scrap of paper and this gives me endless trouble when I come to assemble my work.

One final word: the fundamental rule of computational work is that you must never work with figures that might be wrong. You must check your work at each stage before you go on to the next. Checking is a bore and nobody likes it, but one day you will find some obvious error and may have to spend several hours looking for it. Then you will decide that it pays to check as you go along. There is an art in devising simple automatic checks, and a good text-book will be very helpful.

'Writing-up' and Style

In my experience, this is the hardest part of my research. Interviewing and investigating patients is my job and I like it. Although the computing of results is a routine, it is exciting to see the results of one's efforts; but writing it all out! The only suggestion I can make to ease the labour is that you start your writing as soon as you have finished looking through the literature and planned your experiment.

Concerning style of writing, there can be no argument about matters of taste, so what I have to say here is merely an expression of personal likes and dislikes. I believe that the essence of good style in scientific writing is clarity and simplicity. One should write in such a way that the flow of thought in the mind of the reader is easy and continuous. A given sentence might appear clumsy at first sight, but if it presents the ideas in the correct order, so that they are understood easily, it is doing its job. To illustrate what I mean, and to show you also that I practice what I preach, here is an example from Lecture 11. It is for you to decide whether this is a good example or a bad one to illustrate better what one should avoid. The sentence as written is, ' The usual method of measuring blood pressure depends upon the judgement of the observer of the moment of appearance of certain sounds in the stethoscope, or their disappearance or change in quality'. The sentence would be better English if it went as follows, ' The usual method of measuring blood pressure depends upon the judgement of the observer of the moment of appearance, disappearance or change in quality of certain sounds in the stethoscope '. Most people will agree that a high-flown ' literary ' style is rather out of place in a scientific report and may look ridiculous. It is the custom nowadays to write in an impersonal style, but only too often it tends to be deadening. Avoid proxility; you should follow the principle: cut it down, or out.

Avoid popular and fashionable slang. You should write on the assumption that your work will be read many years later and few things sound sillier than out-of-date slang. Already I am tired to death of 'communication', 'multidisciplinary' and 'research-wise'. I remember sitting-in once on an interview for the appointment of a senior registrar in medicine. The candidate assured the Committee that he had had a 'wide spectrum' of experience, based on a 'wide spectrum' of teaching in his medical school. He was firmly convinced of the need for a 'wide spectrum' of tests for the investigation of patients. The only thing that he had never considered was that a person who had had the benefits and privilege of a university education might have a 'wide spectrum' of vocabulary. Make sure you really understand the words you use: 'alibi' means 'elsewhere' not 'excuse'; 'hypothecate' means 'to pawn', not 'to hypothesize'. A 'parameter' is a constant, and describes a characteristic of a population. You can, therefore, never measure a parameter, what you measure are 'variables'. Please do not write 'feel' when you mean 'think', 'believe', 'consider', 'suggest', 'propose' or 'guess'. If you are writing in English, try to avoid splitting your infinitives (this is standard in the American language). Finally, when you have written something, let it lie fallow for a few days at least and then revise it. If you can persuade a candid friend to read it and criticize, so much the better.

Summary

This lecture has consisted largely of advice on simple routines for handling the data from experiments. Data are very precious and it is easy to get them into a muddle and even to lose them; a proper routine is a small matter but it will simplify your work and render the task of computing easy. If things go wrong at this stage, the results can be disastrous.

Finally, I have taken the opportunity to air some of my prejudices on the writing of scientific papers. Since I am a consumer of this product, as we all are, I am entitled to some opinions on it, but as doubtless you have your own, you need not take my advice on the subject.

I hope that these lectures will have encouraged you to march cheerfully into the muddy field of clinical research. May I wish you every success.

Tests of Statistical Significance

This lecture may be regarded in a sense as a postscript. In the course of previous lectures I have referred to methods of statistical analysis and even described some in detail. Others I have mentioned or hinted at. For the sake of completeness, I am now going to describe some of these other methods but as these lectures are not intended to be a course on statistics, I shall continue to add comments of clinical relevance.

Goodness of Fit

The first test of statistical significance that I shall describe is one that is simple and has wide applicability. It is used when the criterion is not a quantitative variable, but consists of a set of two or more categories. In other words, the result of the experiment is determined by counting heads. Once again, I will start off with a specific example. One of the reasons why duodenal ulcer is called a psychosomatic disease is because perforation of such an ulcer can be precipitated by emotional stress. It has also been said, among other things, that in this condition anxiety will give rise to pain or exacerbate it. In the course of an investigation on the subject, I decided to inquire about it as it seemed to me that the evidence available was inadequate. There is one difficulty, however. It may well be that, in the course of time, as the condition becomes more chronic, the disturbance of gastric function that shows itself as pain may become sensitive to emotional stress, presumably by some sort of ' conditioning ' process. In other words, the sensitivity of pain to emotional tension is a secondary phenomenon rather than a primary one. If that were so, it would follow that the longer the history of duodenal ulcer, the more likely would the patient observe that ' worry ' gave rise to pain.

The result of my inquiry is shown in Table 15.1. I have abbreviated the original table a little, to make it clearer. Examination of the table shows that among the 96 patients who stated that their symptoms were increased by worry, there were more with a long history of illness than with a short. Conversely, among the 54 patients whose symptoms were not sensitive to worry, there were more with a short history than with a long. These figures would appear to be in agreement with the hypothesis that as the illness continues, there is a tendency for patients to shift from the ' insensitive ' group to the ' sensitive ' group. The only difference is that the differences are small.

TABLE 15.1.   *Frequency distribution of patients*

History	Long	Medium	Short	Total
Sensitive to worry	38	31	27	96
Not sensitive	14	15	25	54
Total	52	46	52	150

The null hypothesis is simple. It states that there is no such tendency and that the figures obtained do not differ from what one would expect to get (in the absence of such a tendency), or rather, that the differences from what one could expect to get could have been obtained by chance, the accidents of sampling. It is obvious that we have to put the null hypothesis into quantitative terms, and the first step in this must be to determine what we mean by ' what we could expect to get '.

The argument runs as follows. Since, in 150 patients there are 96 who are sensitive to worry, how many would we expect to find among 52 patients. The answer is a simple proportion sum. If there are 96 in 150, then there will be 96/150 in 1, and $(96/150) \times 52$ in 52, and this comes to 33·3. In the same way, since 54 out of 150 are insensitive to worry, we would expect to find among 52 patients that $(54/150) \times 52 = 18·7$ are insensitive. The total of 33·3 and 18·7 comes to 52·0 (which checks our arithmetic), i.e. the 52 patients are divided into two groups of such sizes that the ratio between them is 96 to 54, which is the ratio found in the total of 150 patients. In this way we complete the first column of a table (and by coincidence the third column too) and by a similar calculation fill in the

TABLE 15.2.   *Distribution according to null hypothesis*

History	Long	Medium	Short	Total
Sensitive to worry	33·3	29·4	33·3	96·0
Not sensitive	18·7	16·6	18·7	54·0
Total	52·0	46·0	52·0	150·0

other columns. Table 15.2 gives the figures of the ' expected ' distribution of patients, on the assumption of the null hypothesis.

Of course, it is not possible to have a fraction of a patient, but
these are only hypothetical figures calculated to have the exact
proportions. The figures we have actually found obviously differ
from them. What we want to know is how often we would obtain
a discrepancy as large as the one obtained, or larger, by chance.
This could be calculated directly but in practice this would be very
laborious, so the statistician uses an approximation which is
sufficiently accurate for general purposes. The distribution he uses
is the χ^2 distribution (pronounced k-eye square), and the probabilities can be found in the tables in text-books.

The next step is to obtain the discrepancy between the figures
actually obtained and the ' expected ' figures. This is done by subtracting the six entries in Table 15.2 from the corresponding one
in Table 15.1. The result is shown in Table 15.3.

TABLE 15.3. *Differences between ' expected ' and*
' obtained ' frequencies

History	Long	Medium	Short	Total
Sensitive to worry	4·7	1·6	−6·3	0
Not sensitive	−4·7	−1·6	6·3	0
Total	0	0	0	0

The rows and columns of this table add up to zero. Let us
consider why this should be so. If you look at any column in the
table of ' expected ' results, you will see that it adds up to the same
total as the corresponding total in the ' obtained ' results. Then,
by however much one of the two figures differs from its corresponding figure, the other will differ in the opposite direction, thus
bringing the total to the same. It is clear that we could have econo-
mized some labour, for once having found one of the figures in a
column, the other could have been found by subtracting it from
the total. The same would apply to the figures in either of the
remaining two columns. At this point, we can see that each row
has two entries completed, and obviously, we can find the third
entry in the row by subtracting the two already found from the
total. In other words, of the six entries in the table, only two need
be calculated, as the others can then be found by subtraction, i.e.

the remaining four figures are determined by the first two. Try it yourself. In statistical language, this table has two degrees of freedom. In general, any such table has degrees of freedom which can be obtained by multiplying one less than the number of rows, by one less than the number of columns. In this case, there are three columns and two rows, so we obtain the degrees of freedom by multiplying $(3-1) \times (2-1) = 2$.

The six differences measure the total discrepancy from the 'expected' results. We cannot add them together to get a total discrepancy, because they come to zero, some being positive and others being negative. You will not be surprised to learn that the statistician gets over this difficulty by squaring each figure.

TABLE 15.4.   *Differences (deviations) squared*

22·09	2·56	39·69
22·09	2·56	39·69

Here we must pause a moment. Suppose we had got exactly the same sort of results but with twice the number of patients. The discrepancies would then have been twice the size, and the squares would have been four times as big. The total of squared discrepancies increase with the increase in the number of cases, but intuitively, it would seem that it increases too rapidly. Now statistics cannot depend on intuition, but I am not going to give you the mathematical proof that the correct way to handle this problem is to determine the ratio of the squared discrepancies to the expected values. Suffice it to say that the next step is to divide each squared discrepancy by its expected value.

TABLE 15.5.   *Proportionate squared deviations*

			Total
$\dfrac{22 \cdot 09}{33 \cdot 3} = 0 \cdot 66$	$\dfrac{2 \cdot 56}{29 \cdot 4} = 0 \cdot 09$	$\dfrac{39 \cdot 69}{33 \cdot 3} = 1 \cdot 19$	1·94
$\dfrac{22 \cdot 09}{18 \cdot 7} = 1 \cdot 18$	$\dfrac{2 \cdot 56}{16 \cdot 6} = 0 \cdot 15$	$\dfrac{39 \cdot 69}{18 \cdot 7} = 2 \cdot 12$	3·45
Total 1·84	0·24	3·31	5·39
$\chi^2 = 5 \cdot 39$ D.F. $= 2$ P $< \cdot 10$			

The total of the columns comes to 5·39, and this is checked by adding up the rows. This total is known as χ^2, and the probability of obtaining such a figure, or larger can be found by looking up the tables, in the row corresponding to 2 degrees of freedom. The probability is found to lie between 5 per cent and 10 per cent, and this is usually written as $\cdot10 > P > \cdot05$, which means that $\cdot10$ is greater than P which is greater than $\cdot05$. This then is the probability of the null hypothesis and we conclude that there is insufficient evidence to suggest that the passage of time tends to increase the responsiveness of pain in duodenal ulcer to emotional stress.

This test of statistical significance is very useful in many situations. Obviously, it applies whenever our results cannot be described in terms of quantities, but only in different categories, e.g. success or failure of response to treatment; good, indifferent and bad results; died and survived. It can also be used when we have quantitative measures, but there are not enough cases for using the full data. In the above example, the length of history was available in terms of length of years, but there were many particular years, and even groups of years, for which no patients were available. It was therefore more convenient to group the length of history into three categories. Finally, since the test is not based on any underlying assumptions about the distribution of your data, it can be used when the data has a distribution that is anything but Gaussian.

Student's t Test

The next example compares the difference in the effects of two treatments given to two groups of patients, one given ' intensive rehabilitation ' and the other given ' routine care '. The scores are difference-scores on a rating scale of symptoms. The patients were assessed at the start of the trial and at the end and the final score was subtracted from the initial score. The analysis of variance is shown in Table 15.6. Notice that the deviance within groups is calculated directly and also obtained by subtraction. This serves as a check on the calculations. The results are significant at the $\cdot025$ level and the null hypothesis is rejected. We accept the hypothesis that I.R. produces a significantly higher improvement score than R.C. The test of significance merely tells us that we can reject the null hypothesis but does not tell us how much better is one treatment than the other. The data gives us information on this. In round figures, the between-groups deviance is 851 and the total deviance is 10,000, so the between-groups deviance accounts for $851/10,000 = \cdot0851$ or $8\cdot5$ per cent. This is only a small effect.

TABLE 15.6.   *Analysis of variance—two groups*

	Group I.R.	Group R.C.	Total
Number of cases	27	36	63
Total score	502	402	904
Mean	18·5926	11·1667	
Crude sum of squares	13,286	9,686	22,972
Deviance	$13,286 - 502^2/27$ $= 3,952 \cdot 5185$	$9,686 - 402^2/36$ $= 5,197 \cdot 0000$	$9149 \cdot 5185*$

Sums of squares for:

Total	$22,972 - 904^2/63$	$= 10,000 \cdot 3175$
Between groups	$502^2/27 + 402^2/36 - 904^2/63 =$	$850 \cdot 7990$
Within groups	$10,000 \cdot 3175 - 850 \cdot 7990$	$= 9,149 \cdot 5185*$

Analysis of variance

Source	D.F.	Sum of squares	Mean squares	F	P
Between groups	1	850·7990	850·7990	5·67	<·025
Within groups	61	9,149·5185	149·9921		
Total	62	10,000·3175			

Most textbooks compare the difference between two groups by means of Student's t test, largely for historical reasons, as the t test was developed many years before analysis of variance. The layout of this test is shown in Table 15.7. The first five rows are the same as in the previous table. We calculate the variance of the population by dividing the within-groups deviance by its degree of freedom 61 and the answer comes to $V = 149 \cdot 9921$. The variance of the mean of group I.R. is $V/27$ and of group R.C. is $V/36$ as I described in Lecture 9. The variance of the difference is the sum of the two variances and comes to 9·7195 as shown. The standard deviation of a mean is known as the standard error and so the standard error of the differences is the square root of $9 \cdot 7195 = 3 \cdot 1176$. The ratio of the difference between the means to the standard error of the difference, i.e. putting it in standard units, is known as t and it comes to 2·38 which is significant at the ·025 level. Note that the F ratio in the previous table is 5·67 and the square root of $5 \cdot 67 = 2 \cdot 38$. For two groups $F = t^2$. Since the two tests are based on the same theories about distributions, they give the same answer, though they approach it in a different way. The essential difference is that analysis of variance can be generalized to more than two groups.

The conditions under which these two tests can be carried out are that the different groups should have been drawn at random and independently from the same parent populations, i.e. they can be regarded as random samples. This applies also after the treatments, but in practice, this is guaranteed by random allocation to treatment. The variance of the criterion measures should be the

TABLE 15.7. *Student's t test*

	Group I.R.	Group P.C.	Total
Number of cases	27	36	
Total score	502	402	
Mean	18·5926	11·1667	
Crude sum of squares	13,286	9,686	
Deviance	3,952·5185	5,197·0000	9,149·5185
Degrees of freedom	26	35	61

Variance of population$=V=9{,}149\cdot5185/61$
$$=149\cdot9921$$

Variance of Means   Gr. I.R. $149\cdot9921/27$
      Gr. R.C. $149\cdot9921/36$

Variance of difference between means$=149\cdot9921/27+149\cdot9921/36$
$$=149\cdot9921\,(^1/_{27}+^1/_{36})$$
$$=9\cdot7195$$

Standard error of difference$=\sqrt{9\cdot7195}$
$$=3\cdot1176$$

$$t=\frac{\text{Mean}_1-\text{Mean}_2}{\text{S.E. of Difference}}\quad=\quad\frac{18\cdot5926-11\cdot1667}{3\cdot1176}=2\cdot38$$

$$P<\cdot025$$

same for all the treatment populations, which means that the treatments have not affected the variances. The criterion should have a normal distribution in each of the treatment populations, but in practice, the tests give reasonably accurate results unless the distributions are very different from normality. When these three conditions are met, the only explanation for high values of F or t is the differences between the means. A good statistical text will describe how the 'homogeneity of variances' is tested, but it is usually considered to be too sensitive. Only when the variances differ very much should this problem be considered seriously. As for the distributions, the way to examine them has already been described.

How Many Cases?

Suppose that we had laid down before the experiment began that we would require a test of significance to be at the 1 per cent level. We have obtained a P<·025 with 62 patients (rather a large number for a trial run). How many would be required to give us P=·01? The method of work is shown in Table 15.8 and to make the problem more difficult we shall decide to retain the proportions of 3:4 in the groups. In the fraction which gives t, there are four numbers: the difference between the means, the variance of the population and the number of cases in the two groups. We shall assume that the two figures obtained from the experiment remain the same, i.e. in round numbers, the difference between the mean stays at 7·4 and the variance of the population at 150. First, we re-arrange the fraction that gives t so as to leave clear the number of cases. For P=·01, t should be 2·659 and this gives us new equation in which we have replaced the denominator of 108 with C. The solution is C=134·6. The numbers of cases required are therefore 4/135=1/34 and 3/135=1/45, so the sizes of the groups must be 34 and 45, a total of 79 cases. We shall need 16 more cases, 7 for group I.R. and 9 for group R.C. To complete the experiment we would select 16 more cases, randomly allot them into 7 and 9 and carry on with the trial.

TABLE 15.8.   *Estimation of numbers required*

$$t = \frac{7 \cdot 4259}{\sqrt{(149 \cdot 992)(^1/_{27} + {}^1/_{36})}}$$

$$= \cdot 6063 / \sqrt{(^1/_{27} + {}^1/_{36})}$$

$$= \cdot 6063 / \sqrt{(^7/_{108})}$$

$$= 2 \cdot 38 \qquad \text{D.F.} = 61 \qquad P < \cdot 025$$

For P=·01, t=2·659

$$t = 2 \cdot 659 = \cdot 6063 / \sqrt{(^7/c)} \quad \text{where } c = \text{number of cases required}$$

$$c = (2 \cdot 659 / \cdot 6063)^2 \times 7$$

$$= 134 \cdot 6 \backsim 135$$

$$^4/_{135} = {}^1/_{34} \text{ and } {}^3/_{135} = {}^1/_{45}$$

Numbers required are 34 and 45, Total 79.

Analysis of Covariance

In the previous analysis, we used difference-scores as a criterion. We could have used final scores or ratio scores and these would have been analysed in exactly the same way. When we carry out an analysis of variance on the final scores, we recognize that the

TABLE 15.9. *Analysis of covariance I*

Initial score $= X$ *Final (criterion) score* $= Y$

	Group I.R.		Group R.C.		Total	
	X	Y	X	Y	X	Y
No of cases	27		36		63	
Total score	1,034	532	1,211	809	2,245	1,341
Mean	38.2963	19·7037	33·6389	22·4722		
Crude sum of squares	45,996	13,874	45,899	24,197	91,895	38,071
Crude Sum of cross-products	23,292		30,205		53,497	

Corrected sum of squares X

Total $\qquad 91,895 - \dfrac{2,245 \times 2,245}{63} = 11,894 \cdot 6032$

Within groups $\quad 45,996 - \dfrac{1,034 \times 1,034}{27} + 45,899 - \dfrac{1,211 \times 1,211}{36}$
$$= 11,559 \cdot 9352$$

Corrected sum of cross-products XY

Total $\qquad 53,497 - \dfrac{2,245 \times 1,341}{63} = 5,710 \cdot 5714$

Within groups $\quad 23,292 - \dfrac{1,034 \times 532}{27} + 30,205 - \dfrac{1,211 \times 809}{36}$
$$= 5,909 \cdot 5093$$

Corrected sum of squares Y

Total $\qquad 38,071 - \dfrac{1,341 \times 1,341}{63} = 9,526 \cdot 8571$

Within groups $\quad 13,874 - \dfrac{532 \times 532}{27} + 24,197 - \dfrac{809 \times 809}{36}$
$$= 9,408 \cdot 6018$$

Within groups regression coefficient $= b = \dfrac{5,909 \cdot 5093}{11,559 \cdot 9352}$
$$= \cdot 5112$$

Adjusted sum of squares of Y

Total $\quad 9,526 \cdot 8571 - \dfrac{(5,710 \cdot 5714)^2}{11,894 \cdot 6032} = 6,785 \cdot 2250$

Within groups $\quad 9,408 \cdot 6018 - \dfrac{(5,909 \cdot 5093)^2}{11,559 \cdot 9352} = 6,387 \cdot 6246$

final scores are determined by the effects of treatment and also by ' random ' variation. In the analysis of covariance, we also take into consideration the fact that the final scores may be influenced by the initial scores. By ' taking out ' the effect of the initial scores, we are left with what would have been the final scores had all the subjects originally had the same initial score (at the mean). We start with a preliminary triple analysis, see Table 15.9. We divide the deviance of the initial (X) scores into total and within-groups deviances as we do also for the final (Y) scores. Finally, we do the same for the covariance. This follows exactly the same procedure as the analysis of variance but instead of multiplying each X score by itself or each Y score by itself, we multiply each X score by its corresponding Y score. This gives us a total sum of products and a within-groups sum of products. Notice that the within-groups sum of products is larger than the sum of products for total. Variances must always be positive, but covariances can be negative.

The next step is to eliminate from the sum of squares of the criterion scores the effects of the initial scores and this is done as shown in Table 15.9. Thus, we obtain an adjusted sums of squares for criterion scores, both for total and within-groups. We obtain the adjusted sum of squares between groups by subtraction. The reason for doing this is that the within-groups covariance, and therefore the regression constant, is based on a larger number of degrees of freedom, and is therefore a better estimate. Just as we

TABLE 15.10.   *Analysis of covariance II*

Source	DF	Sum of squares	Mean squares	F	P
Analysis of variance : initial scores					
Between groups	1	334·6680*	334·6680	1·77	N.S.
Within groups	61	11,559·9352	189·5071		
Total	62	11,894·6032			
Analysis of variance : final scores					
Between groups	1	118·2553*	118·2553	·77	N.S.
Within groups	61	9,408·6018	154·2394		
Total	62	9,526·8571			
Analysis of variance : adjusted final scores					
Between groups	1	397·6004*	397·6004	3·73	$<·10$
Within groups	60	6,387·6246	106·4604		
Total	61	6,785·2250			

* By subtraction.

lost a degree of freedom because the deviations of the Y scores from their mean summed to zero, so we lose another degree of freedom because the deviations of the adjusted Y scores from the original Y scores also sum to zero. The final analysis of variance is laid out in Table 15.10.

Let us consider this in detail as shown in Table 15.11. The prediction or regression equation is y=b.x, where b is the regression coefficient and y and x are deviations from their respective means. The best estimate of b is from the within-groups data and is the sum of products divided by the sum of squares of X, WGSPY/WGSSX=5910/11,560=·51. The figures are shown more accurately in Table 15.9. Group I.R. has a mean initial score X of 38·3 which is 38·3−35·6=2·7 above the general mean of the X scores. The predicted final score Y is therefore ·51×2·7=1·4 above the general mean of the Y scores. To discount the effect of the high initial X scores, we subtract 1·4 from the mean final Y scores, so the adjusted mean Y score for Group I.R. is 19·7−1·4=18·3.

We repeat the procedure for group R.C. Its mean initial X score is 33·6 and if we subtract 35·6 we get −2·0, the minus sign of which shows that it lies below the general mean. Multiply this by b, ·51 x−2·0=−1·0, and subtract this from the mean final score and this gives the adjusted mean Y score of group R.C. 22·5−(−1·10)=23·5.

When we carried out an analysis of variance on the final scores, the difference between the means of the groups was 22·5−19·7= 2·8 points; by discounting the effects of the initial scores, the difference between the two means has increased to 23·5−18·3=5·2 points (actually 5·1494) and in addition, the population variance (error variance) which acts as the denominator in the test of significance, has been reduced from 154·2 to 106·5, as shown in Table 15.10. This is about 30 per cent and illustrates what analysis of covariance can do to increase the efficiency of an experiment by reducing the error variance.

The other way of discounting the difference between the two groups in their initial scores is to use difference scores and when this was done, it served to bring out the difference between the treatments much more clearly. The reverse is usually the case. This brings us to the conditions or assumptions which are basic to the analysis of covariance. They are the same as for the analysis of variance, but there are two additional ones: the first is that the regressions within the groups must not differ significantly, i.e. they

TABLE 15.11. *Adjusted means of criterion scores*

	Gr. I.R.	*Gr. R.C.*	*Total*
Mean Initial score (X)	38·2963	33·6389	35·6349
Mean Final Score (Y)	19·7037	22·4722	21·2857

Within groups regression=b=·5112

Adjusted mean Y=Mean Y−b (Group Mean X−General Mean X)

Group I.R. $= 19\cdot7037 - \cdot5112\ (38\cdot2963 - 35\cdot6349)$
$= 19\cdot7037 - \cdot5112\ (2\cdot6614)$
$= 19\cdot7037 - 1\cdot3605$
$= 18\cdot3432$

Group R.C. $= 22\cdot4722 - \cdot5112\ (33\cdot6389 - 35\cdot6349)$
$= 22\cdot4722 - \cdot5112\ (-1\cdot9960)$
$= 22\cdot4722 - (-1\cdot0204)$
$= 23\cdot4926$

Criterion scores
Difference between Means $= 22\cdot4722 - 19\cdot7037 = 2\cdot7685$
Difference between adjusted Means $= 23\cdot4926 - 18\cdot3432 = 5\cdot1494$

---

must be effectively the same; the second is that the regressions must be linear, i.e. they must be represented by the regression equation y=b.x, which is the equation for a straight line. Examination of the original data shows that these assumptions are not met and, in particular, the regression in the group R.C. is curved. For this set of data, it would have been better to have divided up the groups to grades or levels of severity in their initial scores and to have carried out a two-way analysis of variance.

Two-way Analysis of Variance

The data in Lecture 9 and this lecture were obtained from an experiment which was carried out in a two-way factorial design. The first factor consisted of drug treatments, Prochlorperazine (PCP), Trifluoperazine (TFP) and placebo (PLAC), and the second factor were the non-drug treatments of intensive rehabilitation and routine care. The data are difference scores and they are laid out in Table 15.12. The first step is to carry out an analysis of variance of the six cells regarded as six separate groups and the result of this is significant, as shown. It happens, sometimes, that this first test does not yield a statistically significant result, and further analysis as described below, does yield significant results. In that case it is necessary to interpret the latter with caution.

TABLE 15.12.   *Two-way analysis of variance 1*

		Gr. PCP	*Gr. TFP*	*Gr. PLAC*	*Total*
Group I.R.	Number	9	9	9	27
	Sum	124	206	172	502
	Mean	13·7778	22·8889	19·1111	18·5926
Group R.C.	Number	12	12	12	36
	Sum	186	195	21	402
	Mean	15·5000	16·2500	1·7500	11·1667
Total	Number	21	21	21	63
	Sum	310	401	193	904
	Mean	14·7619	19·0952	9·1905	14·3492

Crude sum of squares   22,972

Corrected sum of squares

$$\text{Between cells} = \frac{124^2}{9} + \frac{206^2}{9} + \frac{172^2}{9} + \frac{186^2}{12} + \frac{195^2}{12} + \frac{21^2}{12} - \frac{904^2}{63}$$

$$= 2{,}827{\cdot}4841$$

$$\text{Total} \quad = 22{\cdot}972 - \frac{904^2}{63}$$

$$= 10{,}000{\cdot}3175$$

$$\text{Within cells} = 10{,}000{\cdot}3175 - 2{,}827{\cdot}4841$$

$$= 7{,}172{\cdot}8334$$

Source	*df*	*S.S.*	*M.S.*	*F*	*P*
B. cells	5	2,827·4841	565·4968	4·49	<·005
W. cells	57	7,172·8334	125·8392		
Total	62	10,000·3175			

The next stage is to calculate the sum of squares between columns, i.e. due to drug effects. We now turn the table round sideways, so to speak, and repeat the analysis on the rows. Calculating the sum of squares for rows gives the sum of squares attributable to the effects of the non-drug treatments. The sum of both of these comes to $1035{\cdot}5 + 850{\cdot}8 = 1886{\cdot}3$, which is less than the sum of squares between cells. The difference $2827{\cdot}5 - 1886{\cdot}3 = 941{\cdot}2$ is the sum of squares attributable to the interaction between the drugs and nursing treatment. The degrees of freedom of interaction is the product of the degrees of freedom of the interacting factors. In this case d.f. of drugs (columns) is 2 and that of nursing (rows) is 1, so d.f. interaction is $2 \times 1 = 2$. The results are laid out as shown in Table 15.3, and show that the difference between the effects of drug treatments, nursing treatments and their interaction are all statistically significant. If we divide the respective three sums of squares by the total sums of squares, we find that out of the total variability we can attribute 10·3 per cent to interaction. These are small effects though the total 28·3 per cent is not bad.

TABLE 15.13. *Two-way analysis of variance II*

	Corrected sum of squares
Between cells	$=2{,}827{\cdot}4841$
Between columns	$=\dfrac{310^2}{21}+\dfrac{401^2}{21}+\dfrac{193^2}{21}-\dfrac{904^2}{63}$
	$=1{,}035{\cdot}4604$
Between rows	$=\dfrac{502^2}{27}+\dfrac{402^2}{36}-\dfrac{904^2}{63}$
	$=850{\cdot}7990$
Interaction	$=$ S.S. B. cells $-$ S.S. B. rows $-$ S.S. B. columns
	$=2{,}827{\cdot}4841-1{,}035{\cdot}4604-850{\cdot}7990$
	$=941{\cdot}2247$

Source	df	S.S.	M.S.	F	P
Drugs	2	1,035·4604	517·7302	4·11	<·025
Nursing	1	850·7990	850·7990	6·76	<·005
D × N	2	941·2247	470·6124	3·74	<·05
Within cells	57	7,172·8334	125·8392		
Total	62	10,000·3175			

Statistical Significance

The statistical analyses which end with the determination of the probability of the null hypothesis are generally called tests of statistical significance. These tests are applied to the figures which represent the results of the experiment. What these figures mean in the real world is another matter. When the results are obtained from a clinical trial of treatments, there can be a great difference between statistical significance and clinical significance. The latter is a problem which entails consideration of factors of quite a different nature. One treatment may be better than another, as demonstrated by the test of significance, but if the number of cases in the two groups is very large, the actual difference may be negligible clinically. That is why I have been referring to the percentage contribution to the variability. Compared with tests of significance, this percentage gives a much clearer notion of what the results mean in practice. One treatment may be better than another by the test of statistical significance, but you might well decide that the difference was scarcely worth bothering about. Even if the difference were much larger, the treatment which gave the better results might well be rejected on the grounds that its advantages were counterposed by the presence of greater risks, or the need for greater skill or time in getting it, and so on. This argument would not apply, of course, if we were considering mortality rates, because even a small advantage might mean the difference between life and death for some patient; and that is never negligible. Nevertheless, although statistical significance does not predicate clinical significance, the absence of the former settles the question. If a new treatment cannot demonstrate, on a reasonable number of patients, that it is statistically significantly better than the old treatment, it is unlikely that there will be any point in considering it further.

Errors and their Control

In the term ' error variance ' the word ' error ' obviously does not mean ' mistake '. It refers to the variation between subjects which eventually constitutes the denominator in the test of significance. It is evident that this should be made as small as possible, and much of the practical problems of designing experiments is ultimately concerned with reducing the error variance. I have already mentioned a number of such, e.g. dividing groups of patients into ' levels ', selecting a suitably homogeneous population from which to take our sample, increasing the size of the groups, and I have also described the statistical method of analysis of covariance.

You may remember my describing type 1 error, the interpretation of chance differences as being due to the effects of the treatments. Just as chance may lead to a difference between treatment groups, when there are no differences between treatments, so also chance may minimize the differences between groups even when there is a difference between treatments. This is type 2 error and can be expressed quantitatively as a probability. The probability of not missing a difference when there is one is known as the *power* of a test. In the experiment, we increase the power of the test by increasing the number of the subjects or by decreasing the error variance.

When we consider the different sources of ' error variance ' we follow the general rule that the largest source should be reduced first. The principle that we apply is to consider the 'cost'. For example, when we try to reduce errors of measurement, we can do so by devising a more accurate method or by repeating measurements and taking the average. The former may require apparatus and techniques that are not available, but there are limits to the number of, say, blood samples, that one can take from a patient.

Remember that however much you reduce errors of measurement, this will not affect errors of sampling. This is one of the greatest problems in clinical research, because it effects the applicability of the results to clinical practice. The kind of patients to be seen in a teaching hospital differ from those seen in general hospitals, and these again differ from those seen in general practice. The samples seen in hospital, and therefore those most likely to be used for an investigation, are biased samples, and the only way to avoid this is to go into general practice and do the investigation there.

Errors of sampling occur not only in relation to the selection of patients. The relation between errors of measurement and of sampling can be seen very easily in the case of taking a blood-count. It is desirable that the count should be accurate, but however accurate it may be, it will not compensate for errors in the amount of blood taken; and if the blood be taken incorrectly, it will not be representative of the blood in the circulation, and so on.

Interaction

The results of this investigation show that differences between drug treatments are statistically significant. It is obvious that this is due largely to the difference between the drugs and placebo; but this is an overall statement. It is obviously true when the drugs are given under conditions of routine care but not for patients receiving intensive rehabilitation. At this 'level' of nursing treatment, PCP actually does worse than placebo and TFP does better, though in fact none of the drug differences are significant. Turning now to nursing treatments, the results show that intensive rehabilitation gives greater improvement than routine care and this is statistically significant. There is no doubt about this effect when the patients are not given active drugs, but when they do receive them, although TFP does better and PCP worse, none of the differences are statistically significant.

This then is the meaning of interaction, that we can make no general statements about the effects of drugs or nursing care. The effects of the drugs can be defined only in terms of the nursing conditions and vice versa. In general terms, when interaction is significant then we must state the specific conditions under which any treatment effect occurs. The effect of one factor depends upon the level of the other. This is merely a way of describing the results, but we have to go on from there. We have to consider the nature and meaning of the interaction and what lead it gives for research on the effects of the treatments or factors which have been combined.

Equal or Unequal Numbers?

On a number of occasions I have stated that the number of subjects in the different groups should be equal, and certainly the numbers should be as near equality as possible. Why this should be so is a simple question to which a simple answer can be given, but there is more in it than appears at first sight. First, I shall demonstrate the case for two groups. When we examine the difference between two means, using the t test, we divide this difference by a number which is derived from the variance of the population and numbers of subjects in the two groups. In symbolic terms, this denominator is the square root of $V(1/n_1+n_2)$. Since V is a constant, the size of this denominator will depend upon n1 and n2. Suppose we have 10 cases; we can divide them into two groups consisting of 2 and 8, 3 and 7, 4 and 6, and 5 and 5. If you care to check my calculations, you can confirm that $1/n_1+1/n_2$ comes to ·625, ·476, ·417 and ·400 respectively. For any given number of cases, the denominator will be a minimum, and therefore t will be maximum, when the number of cases is equal. It can be proved that this is not only true for two groups but for any number of groups. The argument therefore applies to the one-way analysis of variance for several groups.

For a two-way analysis of variance, the situation is much more complicated. It is true that for any given number of subjects, the best way to arrange them is to ensure that the cells are of equal size, but when they are not, it is not only a question of reduction of efficiency but also that the method of calculating the various sums of squares becomes inapplicable. Another and very complicated method has to be used and this is so laborious and time-consuming that statisticians have gone to a good deal of trouble to find ways of avoiding this. When only an odd case is missing from one or two cells, then a simple solution is possible. What is done is to replace the missing case by an imaginary one which has a score equal to the mean of the cell into which it is inserted. The calculations are then carried out in the usual way but the degrees of freedom are based upon the number of real cases actually included.

The rule that the numbers in the cells should be equal saves a tremendous amount of labour in calculating the results, but it does so at the cost of losing a great deal of material in the experiment. Let us see how this comes about in practice. Suppose we decide to compare three treatments and include as a second factor diagnostic categories or age groups or different centres at, say, four levels. This gives us 12 cells and we decide to have 5 cases in each, making a total of 60. As the subjects arrive they are given the treatments as planned. When, in due course, one of the cells is completed we carry on with the experiment but ignore further cases that would go into the filled cell. Eventually, the experiment is almost complete except for two or three odd cases and we may have to wait months for them. Meanwhile, we are letting go suitable cases simply because the cells for them are already filled. This is a deplorable state of affairs. Obviously the more subjects we can include in the experiment the better. The right way, therefore, to plan the experiment is to decide beforehand the minimum number of subjects required for a cell and then to go ahead and collect all suitable subjects that appear until the smallest cell reaches the required number. The number of subjects in the cells will therefore be very different and one or two may have many more subjects than the minimum number. Since the experiment has many more than the minimum number of cases it will therefore be that much better. Of course, the statistical calculations are now very laborious but that is what computers are for.

Summary

In this lecture I have described the details of computation of a number of statistical tests. At the same time, I have tried to describe the conditions under which they are used and the information which can be obtained from them. I have little doubt that you have found this lecture very difficult; I can only say that I myself have never really understood statistical tests until I have had to do them myself in order to analyse the results of my investigations. I hope you will find some comfort in this.

REFERENCE

LUBIN, A. (1961). The interpretation of significant interaction. *Educational and Psychological Measurement*, **21**, 807-818.

LIST OF REFERENCES FOR FURTHER READING

1. LINDQUIST, E. F. (1942). *A First Course in Statistics*. 2nd edn. Houghton-Mifflin Company.
2. LINDQUIST, E. F. (1940). *Statistical Analysis in Educational Research*. 2nd edn. Houghton-Mifflin Company.
3. LINDQUIST, E. F. (1953). *Design and Analysis of Experiments in Psychology and Education*. Houghton-Mifflin Company.
4. MARASCUILO, L. A. (1971). *Statistical Methods for Behavioral Science Research*. McGraw-Hill Series in Psychology.
5. RULON, P. J., TIEDEMAN, D. V., TATSUOKA, M. M. & LANGMUIR, C. R. (1967). *Multivariate Statistics for Personnel Classification*. John Wiley & Sons, Inc.
6. BROWNLEE, K. A. (1946). *Industrial Experimentation*. 5th edn. London: H.M.S.O.
7. FREEDMAN, P. (1949). *The Principles of Scientific Research*. London: Macdonald.
8. BRIGHT-WILSON, E. JR. (1952). *An Introduction to Scientific Research*. New York: McGraw-Hill.
9. COX, D. R. (1958). *Planning of Experiments*. Wiley & Sons.
10. FISHER, R. A. (1949). *The Design of Experiments*. 6th edn. Edinburgh: Oliver & Boyd.
11. FISHER, R. A. (1950). *Statistical Methods for Research Workers*. 11th edn. Edinburgh: Oliver & Boyd.
12. BETT, W. R. *The Preparation and Writing of Medical Papers for Publication*. London: Menley & James Ltd.

I would like to make it quite clear that it is impossible for me to mention all the very good books that are available. The few I mention here are those that I myself have read, but of course this does not imply that they are any better than those I have not seen. Some of these books may be out of print, more's the pity.

An excellent little book for introducing the reader to statistical ideas and computational techniques is (1). It is extremely useful to those who find it difficult to add up four figures and get the same answer twice running, but it is a little long-winded for those who have got beyond that stage.

I can recommend strongly (2). This book requires some elementary understanding of statistics, but not much, and it is extraordinarily clear in its explanation of the problems of designing experiments. I found some difficulty in understanding the explanation of analysis of variance and, oddly enough, found that the more advanced textbook (3) was much better in this respect.

These three books are now a little old-fashioned. Current ideas are clearly given in (4), but although the text starts from fundamentals, it cannot be regarded as an elementary introduction to the subject. The title of (5) may appear intimidating and perhaps not relevant to clinical research, but I would urge readers not to be put off. The theme is applicable to the problem of choosing a treatment appropriate to a given patient, and the introduction to the subject is made delightfully smooth and easy.

For those who want a simple guide to some of the principles, and especially to details of computation, I can think of no better book than (6). The difficulty is that very elementary explanations are interspersed among very complex material, which is difficult to understand. Don't be put off, just skip the difficult bits.

An extraordinarily interesting book of a very general kind is (7) and I would strongly urge you to read it, if you can get hold of it. It is not primarily concerned with statistics, being confined strictly to the subject of its title. It is well written and most unusual.

The next book (8) I can recommend strongly. It has set out to do precisely what I have done and has done it a lot better. It covers a much wider ground and can be used as a very satisfactory textbook on statistics. Its only disadvantage to the clinician is that it is written by a chemist, primarily for research workers in chemistry and physics.

On the planning of experiments I can heartily recommend (9), which I found very much simpler than many other books on the subject.

Finally, I most earnestly commend to the reader the two classical works by Sir Ronald Fisher (10) and (11). They are very difficult reading for the beginner, but once the elements of the subject have been mastered, he will appreciate the quality of these two books.

A useful little book on the art of medical writing is (12).

Index

Printed by The Central Press (Aberdeen) Ltd